YOUR
SUPERLIFE

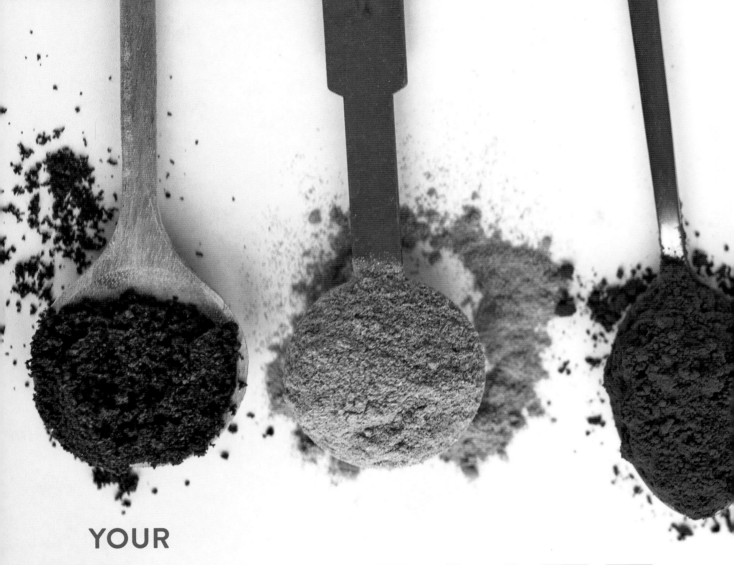

YOUR
SUPERLIFE

Kristel de Groot & Michael Kuech

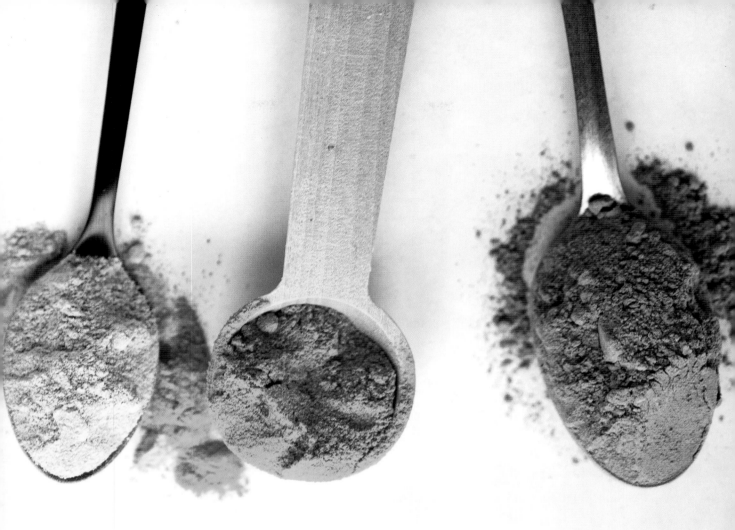

100+ Delicious, Plant-Based Recipes
Made with Nature's Most Powerful Superfoods

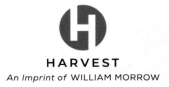

HARVEST
An Imprint of WILLIAM MORROW

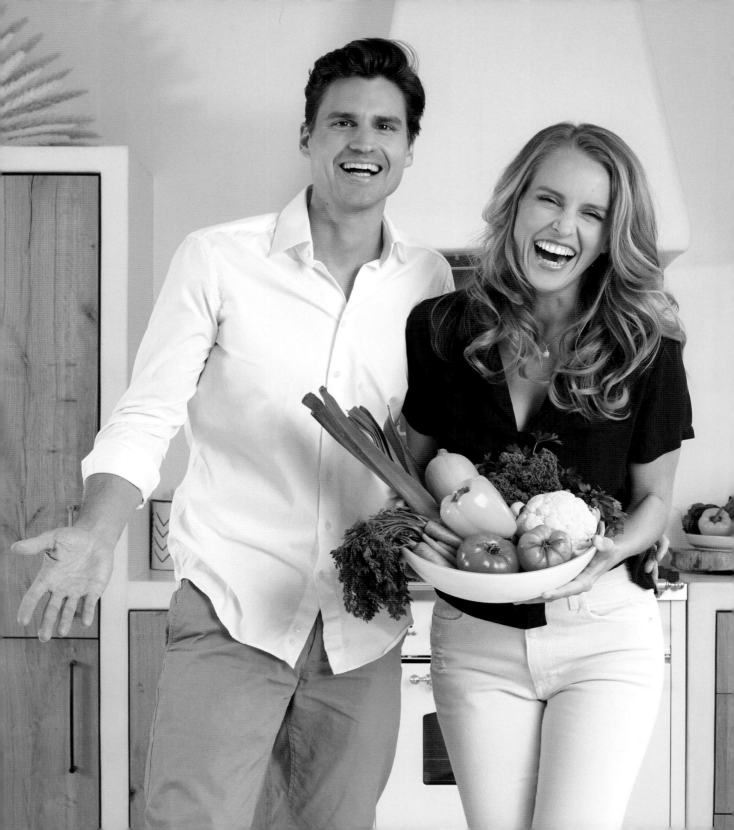

CONTENTS

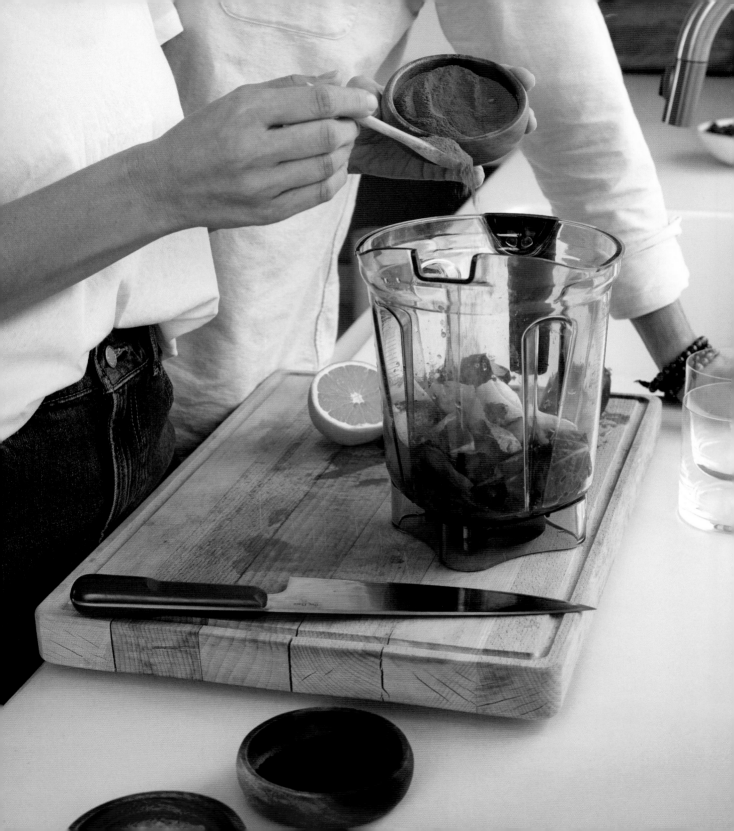

FOREWORD

Anyone who is health conscious is by now aware of the benefits of eating plant-based foods. Mother Nature has imbued plants with natural chemicals called bioactives that interact with the cells in our body. The results of these interactions are powerful, sometimes more powerful than pharmaceuticals, that they are able to deliver their benefits to us three times a day. The power of health therefore lies in the decisions we make each time we sit down for a meal or reach for a snack. *Your Super Life* is a guide to help you make those decisions.

I first met Kristel de Groot and Michael Kuech and after they contacted me to share Michael's story as a cancer survivor. He conquered his cancer with medical treatment, but he restored his health using food as medicine. Kristel and Michael know that good health is not simply the absence of disease—it's something much more than that. When Michael was deemed "cancer-free" by his doctors, he still felt unwell inside. With Kristel at his side, he embarked on a journey back to true health for them both deep into the Amazon rainforest, into wheatgrass fields in Germany, and into the aisles at organic markets where they discovered the power of food as medicine.

In *Your Super Life*, Michael and Kristel share the fruits of their journey by showing you how to eat in a new way. They describe easy steps for changing daily habits that will help your sense of wellbeing. Just as I believe, the path towards better health should focus on what to add to your diet, and not just elimination. Combining all their knowledge of powerful ingredients that they have collected over the years, Kristel and Michael make it easy for you to cook recipes that not only taste good but are easy to make and are packed with foods with bioactives that activate your body's health defenses.

The title of this book *Your Super Life* says it all. There are many remarkable foods with healthful properties, but at the end of the day, there's only one thing that is truly super: your own body. Feed it, nurture it, empower it—and your body will pay you back in spades with years of vibrant health. It's time to start eating the Your Super way.

—William W. Li, MD
New York Times bestselling author of
Eat to Beat Disease and *Eat to Beat Your Diet*

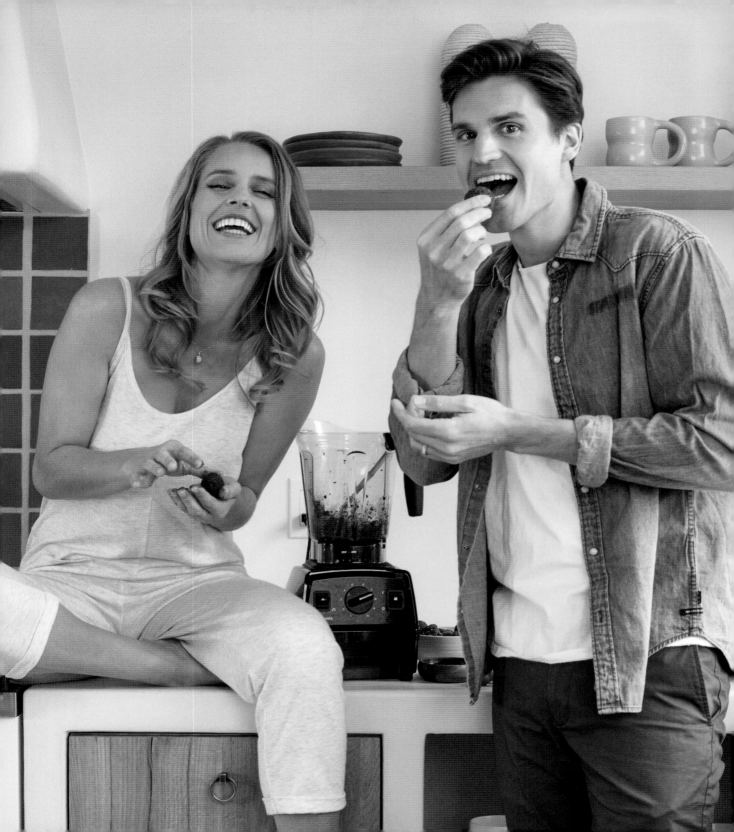

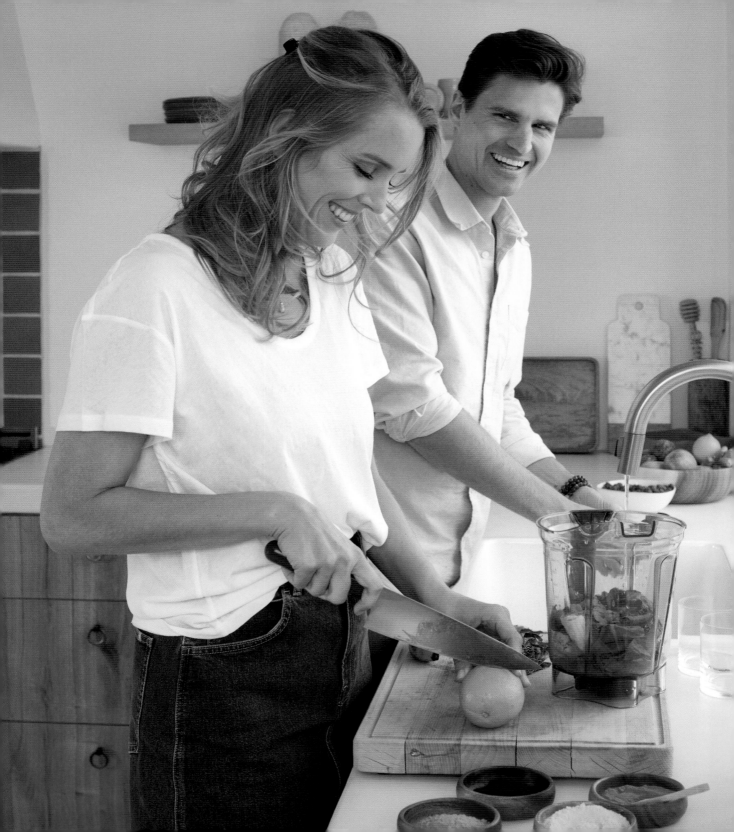

INTRODUCTION

Michael remembers that day like it was yesterday. January 5, 2014. He was twenty-four years old and a former pro tennis player who appeared to be at the pinnacle of good health. It was cold and rainy in Aachen, Germany, and Michael sat on a sterile exam table while the doctor, who was busy scanning him with an ultrasound machine, told him he'd found something suspicious. A few moments later, as Michael sat in his office, the doctor confirmed: It's testicular cancer. Surgery was scheduled for the very next day. Thankfully, surgery and two rounds of chemotherapy removed the cancer from Michael's body. But Michael felt like a shell of himself. "You're cancer-free," the doctor said. "Look at me," Michael responded. He'd lost all his hair. He was the weakest he'd ever felt. But that was it. His doctor had done what he could do. He was fixed.

Michael was relieved that the chemo was effective, but he was also scared. He kept wondering, "Why me?," especially late at night when he was unable to sleep, which was most nights. He became obsessed by this existential question; he was so young and had felt invincible before. He thought he'd been healthy. Why did he get sick? And, even more so, he wondered: "Why does anyone get cancer in the first place?"

The only thing Michael knew definitively was that he never wanted to get sick like this again. So he started to do some research on cancer prevention. What he found shocked him. Did you know that in 2018, the World Health Organization (WHO) concluded that between 30 percent and 50 percent of cancers can be prevented by avoiding risk factors like smoking, consuming alcohol, and exposure to indoor and outdoor air pollution, and by implementing prevention strategies such as regular physical activity and eating a healthy diet full of fruits and vegetables?[1] An earlier report found that up to 30 percent of cancers are linked to poor dietary habits and advised consuming a diet that emphasizes plant foods.[2] In other words, the food we eat can be a powerful tool to help prevent cancer.

But it's not just cancer. The WHO also found that a diet low in saturated fats, limited in salt and sugar, and high in fruit and vegetables (at least five portions a day!), lentils and beans, nuts, and whole grains like oats, millet, and brown rice can also help prevent other chronic diseases such as obesity, cardiovascular disease, and diabetes.[3] Michael thought: "This is it. I might not be able to control all my risk factors related to cancer and other chronic diseases, but I *can* control what I eat. I can absolutely make sure I fuel my body with the best possible nutrition in order to minimize the risk of going through this again." In that moment, Michael stopped feeling scared and started feeling empowered. He could do this.

The Seeds of Change

Michael didn't yet know *how* he was going to do it, but he knew he was ready to make a major change in the way he ate. Luckily, he had Kristel, his college sweetheart, to guide him. Ever since they'd met five years earlier, Kristel had been the resident health nut in his life. He was pretty sure she could help.

While it's true that Kristel was the only person Michael knew who'd bring thick, bright green smoothies to her morning classes during grad school in London, her relationship with food, health, and her body had its own complicated history. Kristel first made the connection between food and wellness years earlier, when she was ten or eleven years old. From infancy, she'd suffered from very bad, painful eczema. For years her mom tried to figure it out, carting her from doctor to doctor and hospital to hospital and trying holistic solutions as well. Nothing

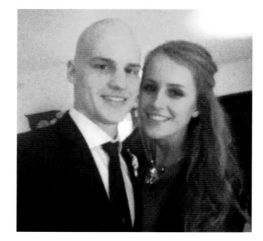

seemed to work. But Kristel noticed that after eating certain foods, like sugar or dairy products, she'd have a bad flare-up. That taught her that there was a relationship between what she put in her body and her skin health.

But this awareness was far from a solution. Kristel came to the United States for college in the early 2000s and, like most first-year college students, gained a lot of weight. She bought into the idea that she *had* to be skinny. Food was her enemy. She did all the popular diets, everything from low-carb to that lemonade-with-cayenne thing. She read her first plant-based-diet book during this time: Kris Carr's *Crazy Sexy Diet*. Kristel was intrigued by the purported health benefits of plant-based foods and the way they supported detoxing your body, but still found herself in an endless cycle of trying the next new thing that promised to help her lose weight and always stressing about and monitoring her food. Meanwhile, despite all the health crazes she was attempting, her eczema continued to cause her pain. During good times, she could keep it managed with a steady stream of antihistamines and steroid creams. During bad times, she'd have painful, itchy rashes all over her face, chin, neck, arms, wrists, and even behind her knees, despite the medicine and creams.

She hit rock bottom at age twenty-two as she was finishing her master's degree. After years of extreme cycles of not eating, feeling depressed, and then overeating until feeling sick, she decided enough was enough. And then, Michael was diagnosed with cancer. For Kristel, Michael's diagnosis was a wake-up call. Her mom had had cancer when Kristel was twelve years old and now Michael—she wanted to do anything she could to reduce her own chance of getting cancer and to help Michael stay in remission. Kristel also realized that Michael wasn't *healthy*, he was *cancer-free*—and there was a difference.

Our Super Life Journey

Together, we decided we'd start doing things to get us *both* healthy.

Our lives were forever changed when we watched the movie *Forks Over Knives*. This film introduced us to *The China Study*, a historic decades-long research project that tracked thousands of individuals in China and found that cancer growth can be turned on and off based on what you eat, and that consuming animal protein is associated with more chronic disease.[4] This seemed like the answer we were looking for: a way to bolster health and immunity and prevent disease. We went plant-based the very next day.

MOVIE NIGHT!

Check out Michael and Kristel's favorite documentaries to learn more about why a plant-based diet is so beneficial for so many reasons:

What the Health

Forks Over Knives

The Game Changers

Cowspiracy: The Sustainability Secret

Seaspiracy

David Attenborough: A Life on Our Planet

Earthlings

Food, Inc.

The first thing Kristel did was put us both on a detox. Then, with the help of her mom and aunt, who are both orthomolecular nutritionists, she created superfood mixes and immune-boosting meal plans that included green juices, nutrient-rich smoothies, and clean, plant-based meals to support Michael's recovery from his chemo treatments. Kristel would drag Michael to Whole Foods, while he complained that this was expensive ("Why does this bag of powder cost forty dollars?!") and complicated ("What the hell is spirulina?!"). She was creating the most powerful and detoxing green superfood mixes for him and insisting, "Whatever you do, take this daily."

All the while, we started to learn more about these superfoods—matcha, wheatgrass, spirulina—that we'd never heard of before, but were suddenly having every day. We were surprised to find that these foods have been around for hundreds—in some cases, thousands—of years, and that people have used these very specific ingredients for functional benefits and food as medicine in many cultures around the world. Wheatgrass contains high doses of chlorophyll, antioxidants, and vitamins A, C, and E, as well as iron, magnesium, calcium, and amino acids. It helps detoxify heavy metals and environmental chemicals, boosts the immune system, calms inflammation, and promotes oxygen levels in the body. It can be traced back more than 5,000 years to ancient Egypt, and perhaps even earlier to Mesopotamian civilizations. It is purported that for ancient Egyptians the young leafy blades of wheatgrass were sacred, prized for their positive effect on health and vitality.

We learned that farmers who grow matcha cover their tea plants twenty to thirty days before harvest to avoid direct sunlight. This increases chlorophyll production, boosts the amino acid content, and gives the plants a darker green hue. Matcha is high in antioxidants, long-lasting caffeine, and L-theanine, which has been shown to increase alpha wave activity in the brain and may help induce relaxation and decrease stress levels. Zen Buddhists in the ninth century used it to help them sit for hours in meditation.

In addition to what we learned about the plant world, we were in awe of what we experienced for ourselves. Michael quickly regained energy and rebuilt his immune system. He was sleeping better and feeling stronger, and his mental health improved too. Kristel's relationship with food began to heal as well. She discovered that plant-based eating allowed her to experience total food freedom; she could eat as often and as much as she wanted, and she felt better and her body came to a healthy weight without deprivation or her tracking what she ate. Her depression lifted. She came to understand that food is not the enemy; it is the world's oldest and most potent medicine. She learned not to fear food, but to embrace it. She stopped stressing about how much she was eating and started eating intuitively, eating much more than she ever did before.

Having experienced these benefits, Kristel wanted to take her healing journey even further. She started incorporating powerful herbs called adaptogens that could support hormone health, like shatavari, which has been used for many year in the Ayurvedic tradition as a support for PMS, infertility, pregnancy, and even menopause. Soon her period pain eased too.

Then about two years into her plant-based journey something unexpected happened: Kristel's eczema completely went away. Eating a whole-food, plant-based diet decreased her inflammation and healed her gut. By no longer putting things in her body that were making her sick, she was able to stop taking all the eczema supplements and prescriptions she'd been taking her whole life and live eczema free.

Ancient Healing for Modern Times

Throughout our healing journeys, we learned so much about the healing properties of plants and what nature can do for our health and well-being. We learned how to combine certain ingredients to create supercharged foods for recovery and healing. We also quickly realized that we weren't alone in our desire to improve health, ward off disease, and enjoy the incredible benefits of nature's medicine. There were countless others just like us—people who want to be healthy but don't know where to start, are confused by the world of superfoods, and are dissuaded by the high prices they see in food markets. That's why we started Your Super in 2014—to make superfood mixes easier to understand, access, and use and to make healthy eating simple and delicious.

SUPERFOOD SUCCESS STORY

ASHLEY

For years I struggled with severe irritable bowel syndrome (IBS)—cramping, bloating, gas, abdominal pain, and constipation. I was a vegan, but not a healthy one. When I finally decided to switch to a whole-food, plant-based diet, Your Super mixes helped me focus on adding the extra nutrition my body needed. I used the mixes that contained wheatgrass, moringa, baobab, spirulina, chlorella, turmeric, tulsi, and ginger. It seems impossible but my IBS symptoms went away overnight. My stomach aches went away. I was regular for the first time in my entire life. And I had way more energy. I even lost weight, but I was eating more! To someone who struggled with eating disorders from ages fourteen to thirty-two, this was huge. I no longer count calories and now have a healthy relationship with food. I also started running again and committed myself to things I love. I still use the mixes pretty much daily.

We created our superfood mixes together with Kristel's mom and aunt. They have no fillers, and are organic, plant-based, and sustainably sourced. In the very beginning, we were mixing things by hand in an organic-certified room in our house so we were able to see the quality of each superfood and note which were the most vibrant, fragrant, and potent. One wheatgrass we sourced was yellowish and didn't smell like anything, whereas a wheatgrass we sourced from a farmer in Germany was bright green and smelled like grass. As we slowly changed our diet over that first year or two, we spent weekends at farmers markets getting feedback on our mixes. We also expanded our culinary horizons from those early months of eating the same few things—smoothies, some nuts, hummus with broccoli, zucchini, roasted eggplant, and basic salads. We read more cookbooks and learned new recipes. We experimented with vegan-izing our old favorite meals and creating our own new recipes. And we explored creative ways to bring superfood powders into every meal of the day.

In the years since we started this journey, we've had some incredible adventures. We've been to Germany to visit the wheatgrass farm and connect with our supplier, who's been farming it for twenty years. We've slept in hammocks in the Brazilian jungle—we even tried to climb açaí trees as our growers do, but we couldn't do it! We know how hard our farmers work for these ingredients. It's also important to us to know how indigenous people use these ingredients. After all, these superfoods are nothing new; we're simply resharing old information that many other healing modalities, from Ayurveda to Eastern medicine to South American traditions, have been utilizing for thousands of years. Whether it comes to superfoods or our healthy, delicious recipes, inspiration and knowledge are found all around the world from a variety of different traditions and cultures.

We started a website to share our story along with our plant-based recipes and mixes. In the years since 2014, Your Super has taken off. Over the last nine years we have shipped plant-based products to more than 2 million people, and led approximately 500,000 people through our plant-based detox program. The number one question we get after our detox program is "How do I eat afterward?" This book is our answer.

In this book you'll find more than one hundred of our favorite recipes, meals and snacks we eat regularly to support our health and fuel our busy lives. We'll teach you our food philosophy and the principles we follow. We'll show you how to eat a whole-food, plant-based diet that is delicious and easy and will optimize your health and make you feel better than you ever thought was possible.

How to Use This Book

Doctors say "eat more fruits and vegetables" and most people want to do this, but are lost when it comes to getting started. How do you really make healthy eating part of your daily life?

That's where we can help. We've done all the work for you. We want to make it easy to bring delicious plant-based superfoods into your diet to nourish and heal you. That's always been our mission.

This book is here for you, wherever you are on your journey to health. Are you struggling to get more plants into your daily routine? We've got you covered. Do you have a chronic condition or a specific health need? Look no further. Whether you want to boost your energy in the morning, need support to de-stress and rest in the evening, or need hormonal relief, the plant world is here for you. We've spent much of the last decade unlocking the hidden power of plants.

We open the book with everything you need to know about this way of eating and how to get started. In Part 1, we take a deep dive into the myriad healing benefits of superfoods, and explain the variety of ways they can improve your health and overall wellness. As you'll see, the benefits can include:

- Renewed energy and focus
- Weight loss and normalized weight
- Increased immunity
- Better mood
- Improved sleep
- Easier digestion

- Less hunger and fewer cravings
- Reduced inflammation and bloating
- Disappearance of eczema and psoriasis
- Reduced risk of chronic diseases like cancer, obesity, heart disease, diabetes, arthritis, IBS, and Crohn's disease, depression, and more!

We'll also walk you through everything you need to know to get started with this way of eating, including pantry staples and meal plans.

The fun begins in Part 2, where we share more than one hundred recipes to nourish you all day long. We've organized the chapters to correspond to the six natural meal- or snack times:

- Breakfasts that start your day with an uplift in health and energy
- Midmorning snacks to keep you satiated and energized
- Filling and nourishing lunches to support gut health and digestion

- Afternoon snacks that are hydrating and stress-busting
- Cozy, simple dinners to help you recover from your day
- Comforting sweets and treats to support rest in the evening and sleep

In these chapters, we'll share filling, vibrant plant-based meals, drinks, and snacks as well as our philosophy behind why we focus on certain foods and superfoods.

We also know that everyone's health journey and needs are different, and we want to help you find the superfoods that most support you so you can create meals that are individualized for your unique needs. Do you need a boost of energy? Comfort? Calm? Immune support? Hormonal balance? Whatever your needs—and they may shift throughout the day and throughout life—we include different superfood recommendations that you can add to recipes if you want extra superpow(d)ers, like our hormone-balancing Berry Hormone Smoothie or our immunity-boosting Green Super Balls. Each recipe is labeled with its superpowers so that you can customize your diet based on your needs. We label recipes by category:

SUPPORT CATEGORIES

SKIN HEALTH	**ENERGY**
DETOX	**HORMONE HEALTH**
IMMUNITY	**PLANT PROTEIN**
ANTI-INFLAMMATION	**MOOD BOOSTING**
STRESS REDUCTION	**HEALTHY FATS**

Because our goal is not just for you to make the recipes in this book, but for you to learn how to create your own recipes based on your preferences and ingredients, you'll find lots of "How To" guides throughout where we'll show you how to assemble dishes in five easy steps with whatever ingredients you have at home.

If you're transitioning to a healthier, plant-based lifestyle—or are trying to incorporate more plant-based meals into your diet—you'll want to find your new go-to recipes. It's common for people—us included—to make the same five or so dinners and two or three breakfasts over and over again. We're confident you'll find some new favorites in these pages to support you on this path.

HOW TO

MAKE OATMEAL 92	**MAKE A SALAD BOWL 170**
BUILD A SMOOTHIE 96	**MAKE A PASTA BOWL 236**
MAKE PLANT MILK 130	**MAKE A VEGGIE STIR FRY 240**
MAKE POWER BALLS 132	**MAKE A QUICK CURRY 242**
MAKE SOUP 167	**MAKE ROASTED VEGGIES 244**

ASHLEY M.

I was diagnosed with ADHD when I was eighteen years old. I was on this medication for close to ten years, when another doctor told me that among other things, this medication can cause heart damage if taken for too long. This scared me. I wanted to make a change, but wasn't sure what to do. I asked the doctor, but they just wanted to switch me to different meds. I didn't like this answer because each potent drug comes with a long list of side effects. As a nurse working in the ICU, I can't afford any setbacks. I have to be at the top of my game so that I can care for my critically ill patients the way they need me to. Shortly after I became vegan, I found Your Super and started trying their products. When I read about Power Matcha and its potential benefits with energy and focus—two main things I lack with having ADHD—I decided to start the process of weaning off my ADHD medication and supplementing with Power Matcha. I have now been off my ADHD medication for almost two years, and I have Your Super and their wonderful products to thank for that. I still have Power Matcha (along with Super Green and Gut Feeling) every morning, but have since also incorporated a daily latte with Super Brew, Magic Mushroom (hello, brain health!), and Plant Collagen. It feels so good to know that I am fueling my brain, and body, with whole organic superfoods, and am no longer at risk for side effects from the potent stimulant I was taking before.

Our biggest tip for transitioning to a more plant-based and superfood-enhanced way of eating is to keep it simple. You'll see this philosophy reflected in our recipes and the guides throughout this book. We want to make it as easy as possible to bring more healing superfoods and plant-based goodness into each moment of your day. This is what helped us make the shift, and we want you to have our best tips and support on your own journey.

You may be skeptical that plant foods can truly offer so much healing and nourishment, and that's understandable. But think about your own health and how you feel day by day. Do you struggle to have enough energy to get through your daily to-do list? Lack the motivation to exercise? Have trouble sleeping? Have difficulty staying at or achieving a healthy weight? Struggle with negative thinking? Find it difficult to concentrate? If you answered "yes" to any of these questions, then we encourage you to rethink what you eat on a daily basis. Yes, there could be other reasons besides diet for these symptoms, but feeding your body a variety of nutrients in their most natural states (in other words—eating plants!) is one of the easiest and most delicious ways to drastically improve how you look and feel. Even if you don't have any of these symptoms but just want to feel more *alive*, plants are your answer.

That's because animal products and overly processed foods can be difficult for the body to digest and often lack the variety of nutrients your body needs to thrive. When the majority of your diet consists of foods with poor nutritional value, you constantly feel hungry. You could try to "will" your way through ignoring constant hunger pangs, but we know we'd rather use our energy for something else! Consistent hunger leads to snacking, which in turn requires more energy for digestion, which can lead to energy dips . . . so you reach for a caffeinated drink, but then may feel jittery and have trouble concentrating, or you may have trouble falling asleep. Then, you wake up feeling groggy and in a bad mood so you reach for a sugary or carb-heavy breakfast and the cycle continues. Sounds pretty miserable, right?

The cycle I described above may seem harmless, and when done once in a while, it is. But when more days are spent in this unhealthy cycle than not, it's easy to see how our weight spirals out of control, we develop nutritional deficiencies, and we may become more susceptible to all kinds of diseases.

But here's the good news: Plant-based eating breaks the cycle! Just as these seemingly small unhealthy decisions can have disastrous consequences, the reverse is also true. Small healthy decisions—when made consistently—can dramatically improve your health, and they work pretty quickly. When you eat a diet of nutrient-dense, whole foods, you will feel satisfied and have sustained energy throughout the day. No energy crashes, no mood swings, no guilt.

With more than one hundred recipes with plenty of special plant add-ons for your specific needs, guidance on how to eat a healthy plant-based diet and how easy it is, the low-down on why plants are so healing, our favorite ways to cook with fruit and veggies, key staples to have at home, and daily meal plans for you (and your family!), this book has everything you need to know to make plant medicine work for your life. We truly believe you can be healthier and happier, have more energy, and feel better than you ever thought was possible. We've made it our mission to make sure you do!

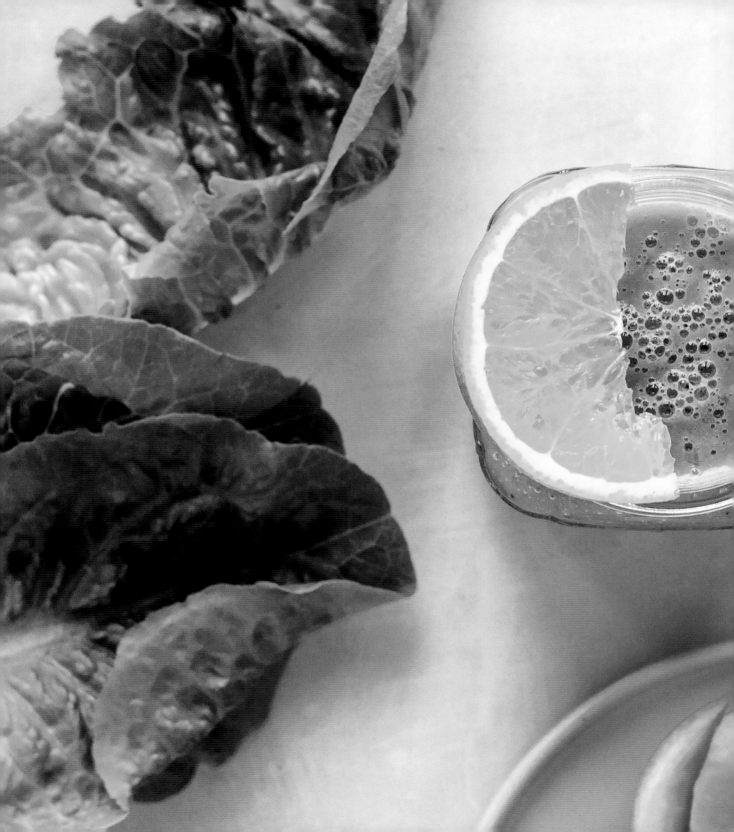

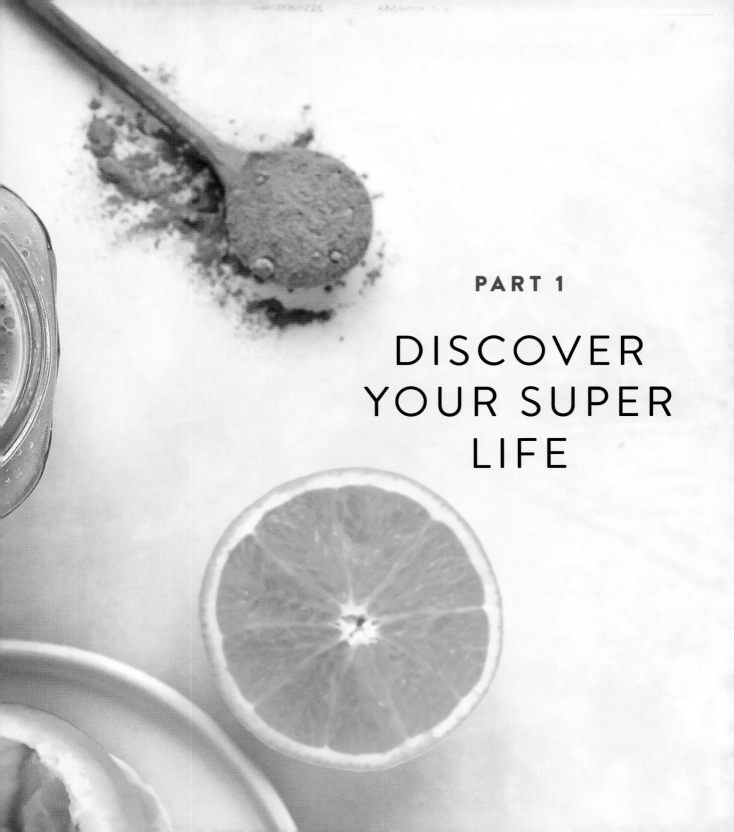

PART 1

DISCOVER YOUR SUPER LIFE

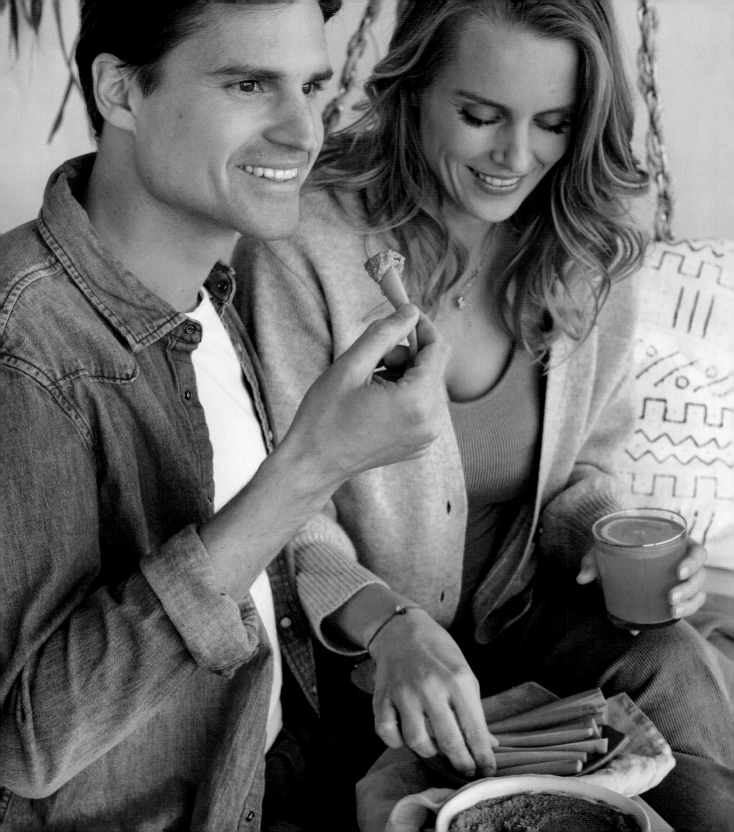

YOUR
SUPER WAY
OF EATING

Plants have so many powerful ways to nourish us: They can help us sleep, balance our blood sugar and our hormones, give us energy, support our digestion, give us healthy skin, detoxify our bodies, nurture our mood and mental health, and so much more. While in the Western world we often think of health as how you look, the Your Super way of eating is about *how you feel*. Do you feel vibrant? Well rested? At ease? Nourished? Do you have energy—the energy to do all the things you want to do? If you follow the Your Super approach to eating, this is how you will feel. It's not a quick fix, but a philosophy of food as medicine that can transform your life.

We want to help you unlock all the power that plants have to heal and take care of you. With just a little knowledge and guidance you can use food to improve your health and feel your best. We want to help you get more connected to how your food makes you feel and help you eat food that loves you back. It doesn't have to be complicated or overwhelming. All the recipes and tips you'll find in the pages to come are based on our simple food philosophy, which has just three pillars:

1. HEALTHY

You want your food to be doing something good for you and to do that you want it to be packed with nutrition. Focus on real whole foods, fruits, and veggies—in short: PLANTS! All the good stuff is found in whole foods and nutrient-dense superfoods. Rather than thinking solely about macronutrients like fat, protein, and carbs, eating whole plant foods will help you get tons of micronutrients—really powerful things like vitamins, minerals, enzymes, phytonutrients, and antioxidants—that are found in real plant foods that will help your body thrive. Try to eat about 50 percent raw, uncooked fresh whole plant foods to optimize the enzymes, vitamins, minerals, and phytochemicals (plant compounds that may fight cancer and other diseases) in your diet. Exclude or limit processed foods, alcohol, coffee, oils, and animal-based products like dairy, meat, and fish. You don't have to go cold turkey. Instead, focus on eating more of the good stuff and you will see that you will start craving the bad stuff less and less.

We've noticed that people often check food labels to find out how many calories or grams of protein, fats, or carbs a food product contains, but it's actually way more important to read the ingredient list. You want to know what is in your food. Can you recognize all of the ingredients? If not, google it. Then decide if you actually want to put it in your body.

At Your Super we believe that eating real foods makes all the difference. We trust that nature knows best and that there are nutrients in fruits and vegetables that work together for our health that we humans don't even fully understand yet. Our recipes will help you add more fresh, organic, and unprocessed whole plant foods into your daily diet, and limit additives and artificial, processed foods.

WHAT A "CLEAN LABEL" MEANS TO US . . .

No sweeteners—like stevia or artificial sweeteners

No flavors—not even the natural ones

No gums or filler, just real foods

In short, only real plant foods that are minimally processed

---

2. EASY

None of us can spend all day preparing food or have endless free time to make complicated dishes that require an hour here, and ten minutes there, and then let it stand for two days to sprout, and then wait another hour before ready. Don't get us wrong: We love sprouted foods and we love the ritual and culture of in-depth food preparation, but it's just not reality for most of us to cook this way most of the time. We all live busy lives and good food needs to be easy enough to fit in your busy schedules.

These recipes are things we quickly whip up in our kitchen regularly. While they are easy enough to make on a daily basis, they are still packed with creative flavor profiles and potent plant-powered nutrition. Our hope is that you'll come to think of them as your staples too—recipes that are so easy and fast, you'll have them on rotation multiple days of the week.

We also want to emphasize that this isn't about counting calories or tracking macronutrients—in fact, we don't want you doing any of that. We encourage you to eat intuitively, listen to your body's hunger and satiation cues, and focus on ingredients instead of nutrition facts. Change the way you think about food: It is much easier to eat healthy foods when you think of our food as self-care, as a way to nurture and care for yourself. This doesn't have to be complicated. In fact, it's anything but. Your goal is simply to listen to your body and let it tell you what it needs at each stage of your day.

3. DELICIOUS

As important as health is to us, nobody eats only for their health, and if food is easy to prepare but doesn't taste good, then what's the point? We are foodies through and through and we want to show you that the myth that eating plant-based means you only eat broccoli and carrots is far from the truth. You can make delicious food that is packed with flavor—sweet, savory, tangy, umami, and more—without relying on artificial ingredients or animal products. Food that is indulgent and satisfying, and is also full of healing properties. Delicious food is central to eating intuitively. When you love what you eat, you'll want to eat more of it!

GIVE INTUITIVE EATING A TRY

Intuitive eating is all about learning to listen to your body. You eat when you are hungry and stop when you are full. Many of us look to experts for the magic answer on what we should be doing instead of trusting our internal wisdom. When you eat intuitively, you practice listening to your body and trusting that it knows what it needs. This might mean that some days you will eat more and other days you will eat less. That's okay. Often the stress we create by following the rules of a specific diet or counting calories only increases our body's main stress hormone, cortisol, which increases fat storage. When you practice intuitive eating, you let go of rigidity around food and give yourself permission to eat in a way that feels good for your body. It can take some time to get in touch with your body, but it's worth it!

Focus on getting a variety of colors and textures and tastes. Let food be a delightful experience for all your senses. Food is an important part of our cultural and communal lives too—the place where the family comes together, a source of emotional support—and our recipes also celebrate this special place that eating has for each of us.

Every recipe in this book takes these three pillars into consideration. We want it to be easy and delicious for you to eat healthy food, and we want you to learn how to listen to your body.

THE YOUR SUPER PILLARS

HEALTHY

1. **Focus on real, whole foods,** with about 50 percent raw, uncooked fresh whole plant foods that are loaded with micronutrients like vitamins, antioxidants, polyphenols, minerals, and more!

2. **Skip the nutrition label and read the ingredient list instead.** Do you know what everything is? Do you want to put that in your body?

3. As much as possible, **exclude animal-based products** like dairy, meat, and fish, and **limit processed foods, oil,** alcohol, and coffee. If that feels overwhelming, focus on adding in whole plant foods and nutrient-dense superfoods rather than excluding anything . . . and over time, you'll find you crave whole foods more and more.

EASY

1. **Focus on quick, twenty-minute meals** that don't take a lot of work. Healthy eating can be super easy. This book will teach you how.

2. **Eat intuitively:** Listen to your body—avoid calorie counting and tracking macros. Eat when you are hungry and stop when you are full. It's that simple. There are going to be days you will eat more and days you will eat less—that's life.

3. There's **no pressure for perfection or deprivation—focus on feeling good**, fueling your body, and finding a sense of joy and fulfillment. Eating this way is all about overloading your body with the good stuff to get all the nutrients your body needs.

DELICIOUS

1. **Eat more color**—your food should be beautiful and full of flavor! Eat a variety of delicious fruit and veggies—there are so many options. And superfoods pack a punch of color as well!

2. **Follow the 80/20 rule**—focus on getting whole plant-based foods 80 percent of the time, and the rest is up to you! Maybe that 20 percent means vegan ice cream, burgers, or pizza; you'll still reap incredible benefits by sticking to plants 80 percent of the time.

3. **Don't feel guilty . . . enjoy what you eat!** Let food be the centerpiece of cultural traditions, celebrations, self-care, and connection.

Why Plant-Based?

There are three main reasons to eat a plant-based diet. The first is that there's strong evidence that a plant-based diet can prevent and even reverse some chronic diseases—everything from heart disease to cancer to Alzheimer's and more. The scientific community has overwhelmingly come to the conclusion that if we eat more fruits and vegetables, we are healthier. Not only are there numerous studies confirming the power of a plant-based diet to reduce the risk of cancers,[1] as we mentioned in the introduction, but also to:

- Reduce inflammation in the body[2]
- Lower one's risk of Type 2 diabetes[3]
- Improve heart health[4]
- Improve cholesterol levels[5]
- Improve cognitive abilities and lower your risk of dementia[6]
- Improve gut health and digestion[7]
- Improve athletic performance[8]
- Reduce arthritis pain[9]
- Renew focus and energy[10]
- Lose weight and normalize weight[11]
- Increase immunity[12]
- Improve mood and mental health[13]
- Improve sleep[14]
- Heal eczema and psoriasis[15]

Plants are really special because they contain many micronutrients. At least nine different families of fruits and vegetables exist, each with potentially hundreds of different plant compounds that are beneficial to health. While we have been encouraged to worry about our *macro*nutrient intake—in other words, how many grams of protein, carbohydrates, and fats we are eating—the real power of nutrition lies in our *micro*nutrient intake, or the minerals and vitamins in our food. The consumption of micronutrients is important to a healthy body.

For example, plants contain thousands of phytonutrients. Phytonutrients (*phyto* from the Greek for "plant") are natural chemical compounds believed to be beneficial to human health, including helping prevent diseases. They are antioxidant and anti-inflammatory. They may also enhance immunity and intercellular communication, repair DNA damage from exposure to toxins, detoxify carcinogens, and alter estrogen metabolism. Whenever we refer to nutrient-dense food we are referring to foods that are high in micronutrients. Eating a variety of types and colors of whole plant foods helps give your body the mix of nutrients it needs. This not only ensures a greater diversity of beneficial plant chemicals but also creates beautiful, colorful meals that truly look as appetizing as they taste.

Fruits and vegetables are high in the micronutrients your body needs to function well, but most of us aren't getting nearly enough. In fact, nine out of ten Americans don't eat enough fruits and vegetables on a daily basis (the CDC recommends one and a half to two cups of fruit and two to three cups of vegetables daily) and therefore aren't getting sufficient nutrients.[16] Across Europe, similar data shows that eight out of ten people do not eat enough fruits and vegetables daily.[17]

SUPERFOOD SUCCESS STORY

JENNIFER

I used to struggle with stress on a daily basis. I am a single mother who works full-time and is always on the go getting everyone to their extracurricular activities every day. Stress was a huge part of my life. It could be crippling at times and many times predicted my day. When I first found Your Super, I focused on the mixes that were said to alleviate stress. I first did a Your Super Detox and then made sure to keep mixes like Magic Mushroom, Golden Mellow, Plant Collagen, and Forever Beautiful in my daily routine. Even though MM and GM have calming ingredients, I take them each morning and each evening. I continue to do a Your Super Detox the first week of each month as well. I use other Your Super mixes too but these are the ones that I feel focus on my anxiety the most. After the detox and about two additional weeks of using these mixes on a daily basis, my anxiety decreased by 75 percent or more. I was no longer nervous about my activities for the day, about work, or about all the extracurricular activities. I felt more at ease and relaxed each morning and each afternoon. I no longer take any kind of antianxiety medication and am only using Your Super to help with anxiety. As long as I take my mixes, I do not fear having to live with anxiety anymore. Using Your Super with a whole-foods, non-processed, and plant-based diet has changed my life 100 percent.

Another way that plant foods are so good for us is that they are the only source of a diverse range of fiber. Fiber is important because it helps regulate your body's use of sugars, helping to keep hunger and blood sugar in check. It's also essential for gut health and a strong microbiome. Children and adults need at least 20 to 30 grams of fiber per day for good health, but most Americans get only about 15 grams a day.

A plant-based diet, or a primarily plant-based diet, helps us address these inadequacies and fuel our bodies with all the healthy goodness we need to thrive! And we help you make it delicious and easy to do.

The second reason we believe in a plant-based diet is that it's also probably the single biggest way we as individuals can reduce our carbon footprint—by more than 50 percent![18] That's a bigger impact than buying an electric car or reducing air travel. Animal farming is the second largest contributor to greenhouse gas emissions (after fossil fuels) and a leading cause of deforestation, water and air pollution, and loss of biodiversity. One acre of rainforest is cut down for cattle farming every six seconds.[19] One pound of meat uses about fifty full bathtubs of water to produce.[20] A plant-based diet is the best diet for the climate—you'll reduce greenhouse gases, land use, water use, and damage to our waterways and support ecological biodiversity. [21,22]

The third reason we believe in a plant-based diet is that it helps end cruelty to animals. Did you know that every year over 70 billion farmed animals are killed for food? A staggering 99 percent of animals consumed as food in the United States are from factory farms.[23] This number doesn't even include fish and other sea creatures. Even if they're raised organically and live better lives, these animals' lives and deaths are quite cruel. Mother cows are still removed from their crying babies to produce organic milk, for example.

If you aren't interested or don't think you're ready to go fully plant-based, that's okay! Eating 80, 90, or 95 percent plant-based is wonderful for your health. Small steps will lead to big results when you start adding more whole plant-based foods and superfoods to your day. We've made it simple for you to do so! We encourage you to experiment, notice how you're feeling, and start adapting recipes to your liking to find what works best for you.

Why Superfoods?

If plants are the heroes of the food world, then superfoods are the superheroes. They're absolutely bursting with nutrition and medicinal properties. Though they are largely overlooked in the Western diet, superfoods have been prized for their healing and medicinal properties for hundreds, or sometimes thousands, of years. They are truly nature's medicine. We love superfoods because they pack a ton of micronutrients into a small package that's so easy to add to smoothies, stir-fries, baked goods, lattes, and so much more. We all need to eat more whole-plant foods, and superfoods are a quick and simple way to add them!

We live in a world with more stress than ever before. We're expected to always be on and connected, whether it's checking emails at night for work, getting constant messages from friends on our phones, or information overload through social media and television. Experts now say that chronic stress—which is linked with everything from poor mental health to inflammation in the body—is becoming a public health crisis.[24] We're also exposed to an astonishing amount of man-made toxins that wreak havoc on our health—since 1950 there has been a *fiftyfold* increase in the production of chemicals, and that's expected to triple again by the year 2050.[25] Industrial toxins are regularly found in newborn babies, in mother's milk, and in drinking water worldwide.[26] Healthy eating is one of our best methods of resisting the strain that stress and toxins have on our bodies. Superfoods are not a cure-all or an instant fix—you'll likely need to integrate them daily over a period of two to four weeks before you start noticing differences. But when combined with a plant-based diet, superfoods help you optimize your diet to best support your health.

The word "superfood" has turned into a buzzword, and, thanks to clever marketing, it's being slapped on just about anything. (Butter? Really?) With all the confusion and misinformation, many people are left wondering: What are superfoods, anyway?

SUPERFOOD SUCCESS STORY

ROBIN

I've been using Your Super foods for a year. I was struggling with extra weight, low energy, and depression. I had just come down with Covid and decided to kick myself into gear with Your Super Detox followed by the Gut Health Bundle to boost my whole system with wheatgrass, chia, açaí, maqui, acerola, maca, pea protein, hemp protein, spirulina, ginger, and tulsi, among other superfoods. My focus was on filling my body with nourishing foods and rebuilding a solid base. This, along with exercise, helped immensely. My digestion improved, my energy shot up, my depression lifted, and I had a newfound outlook and enthusiasm for nutrition and health. I lost weight too and began running again! Your Super mixes made it easy and fun to get essential nutrients and boost my creativity for new food recipes. I still use Your Super today with just as much enthusiasm and continued benefits!

Well, superfoods are foods that have a very high nutritional density. This means that they provide a substantial amount of nutrients like minerals, vitamins, and antioxidants. The high vitamin and mineral content found in superfoods can help your body ward off diseases and keep you healthier. When incorporated into a well-balanced diet, these foods can promote heart health, support weight loss, improve energy levels, and even reduce the effects of aging.

No single food can do it all—but superfoods have a lot of bang for their buck when it comes to nutrient density. Superfoods are rich in:

- **ANTIOXIDANTS:** These natural compounds protect your cells from damage and may lower the risk of heart disease, cancer, and other diseases.
- **MINERALS:** These essential nutrients (think calcium, potassium, iron, and the like) help your body perform at its highest level.
- **VITAMINS:** It's better to get these organic compounds from natural foods—like superfoods—than from supplements.

Superfoods may also be high in:

- **FIBER:** Fiber supports gut health and helps decrease cholesterol, prevent heart disease, and control glucose in Type 2 diabetes.
- **FLAVONOIDS:** Found in plants, flavonoids (once called vitamin P) have anti-inflammatory and anticarcinogenic properties.
- **HEALTHY FATS:** Monounsaturated and polyunsaturated fats, aka "good fats."

Superfoods are highly nutritious, but we want you to know that they're so much more than that. In addition to the many hours we've spent learning about the nutritional properties of superfoods, we've also traveled the world learning from the people who grow and use them in their native ecosystems and taken deep dives into the histories of how these medicinal foods have been used for hundreds, even thousands, of years. Superfoods are nothing new. We're just relearning and reintegrating them into our Western culture. We love superfoods for the ways they connect us to tradition and culture, and we believe that food is its most potent when we understand it in its fullest context, including nutrition science, culture and ritual, and historical significance.

In Senegal and Ghana, for example, you'll see locals walk right up to baobab trees, take the tree's fruit that dries by itself in its shell, squash it, and consume the citrusy powder. These large, thousands-of-years-old trees are never owned by anyone—they're always public property for people who live in the communities. Ancient Incas in Peru consumed cacao as part of love or heart-opening ceremonies, while in the Indian Ayurvedic tradition, turmeric and shatavari have long been used to help women with fertility and hormone balance. The moringa tree in Africa and India is called the "tree of life"; we eat only the leaves, which contain all essential vitamins and minerals, but you can use every part of the tree for nourishment and healing. In the local communities they even use moringa seeds as a kind of antibiotic.

Healing plant foods connect us to the past, to indigenous wisdom, and to our own best expression of health. We want to help you bring this sense of history, community, and well-being into each part of your day, with simple and delicious recipes that uplift, enhance, and nourish you, body and soul.

In this cookbook we want to focus on what we consider to be the top twenty-five superfoods—those that are most easily available in quality form and, most important, best for your health. These include:

AÇAÍ BERRY

Açaí berries are native to the Amazon region. They are half-inch-round fruits that grow on açaí palm trees. Each fruit contains a large seed, which accounts for 60 to 80 percent of the volume of the fruit. Açaí berries boast three times the amount of antioxidants found in blueberries—so they are perfect for supporting your skin health! It takes 20 kilograms of açaí berries to make 1 kilogram of açaí powder. It is easy to forget how nutrient-dense and concentrated superfood powders can be!

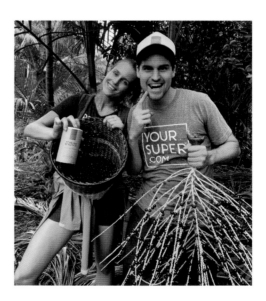

ACEROLA

The acerola cherry is mostly found in South America and Mexico. It is super high in vitamin C, a powerful antioxidant that protects the body against oxidative stress. Acerola has been found to have up to 14.6 milligrams of vitamin C per 1 gram of ripe fruit. This is 50 to 100 times more than is found in an orange! Since they spoil quickly, they're best consumed frozen or in powder form.

ASHWAGANDHA

Ashwagandha is one of the most important herbs in Ayurveda, a traditional form of alternative medicine based on Indian principles of natural healing. It's also known as Indian ginseng. The ashwagandha plant is a small shrub with yellow flowers that's native to India and Southeast Asia. Extracts or powder from the plant's root or leaves are used to treat a variety of conditions, including anxiety. Ashwagandha is an adaptogen—a type of plant that can help your body manage stress.

BAOBAB

The baobab tree grows in low-lying areas on the African mainland, Madagascar, and Australia. It is often owned by the community and only locals are allowed to harvest the fruit. It can grow to enormous sizes, and carbon dating indicates that it may live to be 3,000 years old. Baobab fruit is high in vitamin C, a powerful antioxidant, as well as fiber to support digestive health and balance blood sugar levels. Locals are known to use it for energy as well. The fruit has a hard shell and is already dried within the shell when harvested so it only has to be pulverized to make it into a powder.

CACAO

Cacao has a rich history in Mesoamerican native cultures. Traces of its use date back more than 4,000 years. Cacao gained a sacred status in cultures such as the Olmecs, Izapan, Maya, Toltecs, Aztecs, and Incas. Cacao powder is made from the beans found in the cacao pod. When you open a cacao pod, the beans are surrounded by a delicious-tasting fruit. The bean inside the fruit is purple and extremely bitter.

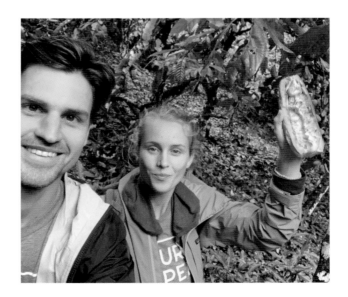

CHAGA

Since the sixteenth century chaga has been used in folk and botanical medicine throughout Eastern Europe. A birch fungus, chaga grows on living trunks of mature birch trees in cold climates. Called the "gift from god" or the "king of herbs," the chaga mushroom has been respected for thousands of years throughout Russia, Korea, Eastern and Northern Europe, the northern United States, the North Carolina mountains, and Canada. Chaga powder is extracted to make the healing compounds in the mushroom bioavailable.

CHIA SEEDS

A staple in the ancient Aztec and Maya diets, chia seeds have been touted for their health benefits for centuries. One ounce (28 grams) has close to 10 grams of dietary fiber. That means they're a whopping 35 percent fiber by weight. The antioxidants, minerals, and omega-3 fatty acids in chia seeds may promote heart health, support strong bones, and improve blood sugar management. They can be eaten raw, soaked in juice, or added to oatmeal, pudding, smoothies, and baked goods. Given their ability to absorb water and fat, you can use them to thicken sauces and as an egg substitute. They can also be mixed with water and turned into a gel. The fiber and protein in chia seeds may benefit those trying to lose weight.

CHLORELLA

Chlorella is single-celled, green freshwater algae that is 60 percent protein. Chlorella has existed since the birth of the Earth and has been reproducing for three billion years. It contains all amino acids and is also a good source of vitamin C, iron, B vitamins, antioxidants, and omega-3. Chlorella can support your body's natural detoxification and immunity.

FLAXSEEDS

Flax is one of the oldest crops, having been cultivated since the beginning of civilization. Its Latin name is *Linum usitatissimum*, which means "very useful flax."[27] Flaxseeds come from the flax plant, which grows to be about 2 feet tall. Flaxseed is rich in alpha-linolenic acid (ALA, omega-3 fatty acid), lignans, and fiber. Flaxseed oil, fibers, and flax lignans have potential health benefits such as reduction of cardiovascular disease, atherosclerosis, diabetes, cancer, arthritis, osteoporosis, and autoimmune and neurological disorders.

GINGER

The known history of ginger dates back about 5,000 years. Its medicinal and spiritual uses were first documented in Southeast Asia, India, and China. Traditional Ayurvedic texts recommend ginger for therapeutic use for joint discomfort; for motion or airsickness; and for clearing the microcirculatory channels to facilitate better absorption of nutrients and better elimination of wastes. Modern science, by way of worldwide research, supports its effectiveness for helping with motion or airsickness, improving digestion, and promoting joint health.

GUARANA

Guarana is also called the edible "eyes of the Amazon." A mature guarana fruit is about the size of a coffee berry and resembles the human eye, with a red shell encasing a black seed covered by a white aril. It has a centuries-old heritage and mythical status for the Sateré-Mawé indigenous people. Its seeds are highly prized for their stimulant and medicinal properties. Numerous research papers explore its potential in the prevention of cardiovascular disease, as an anti-inflammatory, antioxidant, antidepressant, intestinal regulator, and even an aphrodisiac.

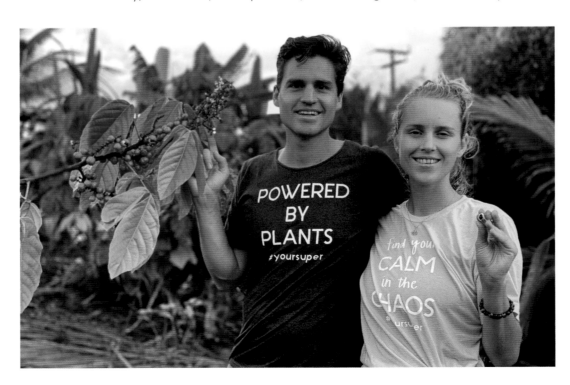

HEMP PROTEIN

Hemp protein is the protein content of hemp seeds. It has an earthy, nutty taste and is often added to shakes or smoothies to boost protein intake. Hemp is a high-quality vegan protein, containing all nine essential amino acids, plus fiber, healthy fats, and minerals. Each ¼-cup (30-gram) serving contains 15 grams of protein. Research shows that 91 to 98 percent of the protein in ground hemp seed is digestible. This means that your body can use almost all of the amino acids in hemp protein powder for important bodily functions, such as repair and maintenance.

KELP

Known as the superfood of the sea, kelp grows in underwater kelp "forests" in shallow oceans and is thought to have appeared in the Miocene 5 to 23 million years ago. The organisms require nutrient-rich water with temperatures between 43° and 57°F (6° and 14°C). It is loaded with iodine, a mineral most of us need more of to support a healthy thyroid.

MACA

Maca root was domesticated around 3800 BCE, with primitive cultivars of maca being found in archaeological sites dating back to 1600 BCE. It continued to be cultivated by the Inca centuries ago as a valuable nutritious dietary staple and adaptogen. Natives of Peru eat up to 20 grams of dried maca daily for their health. Maca is a very nutritionally dense plant and extremely important to overall health in a region where little else grows. Maca is said to increase energy and stamina as well as to boost fertility and libido.

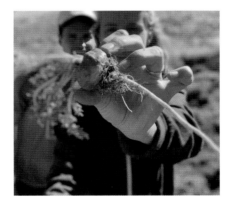

MAQUI

Maqui berries grow wild in South America and are mainly harvested by the native Mapuche of Chile, an indigenous people who have used the leaves, stems, and berries medicinally for thousands of years. Maqui is an even smaller and darker berry than açaí—and it contains even more anthocyanin, an antioxidant compound known for its ability to neutralize free radicals within the body, repair tissue damage, and strengthen the immune system.

MATCHA

Matcha is made of pulverized green tea leaves and was originally used by monks in Japan to better concentrate during meditation. Farmers grow matcha by covering their tea plants 20 to 30 days before harvest to avoid direct sunlight. This increases chlorophyll production, boosts the amino acid content, and gives the plants a darker green hue. Once the tea leaves are harvested, the stems and veins are removed and the leaves are dried and ground into a fine powder known as matcha. Matcha contains the nutrients from the entire tea leaf, resulting in a greater amount of caffeine and antioxidants than typically found in green tea. Matcha has a slower release of caffeine and lower caffeine than coffee—so it gives you around six hours of more stable focus and energy. It creates a calm alertness with just a sixth the caffeine of coffee (25 milligrams versus 150 milligrams in a typical cup of coffee). There are no spikes and crashes; alertness comes on gently and leaves just as gently.

MORINGA

Moringa, a green superfood, was discovered in northern India around 2000 BCE. Traditional doctors quickly discovered its medicinal impact and called it the "tree of life." This herb is one of the most effective and essential medicinal plants in Ayurveda. Moringa contains all essential vitamins and minerals. As an antioxidant, it seems to help protect cells from damage. Moringa may also help decrease inflammation and reduce pain.

PEA PROTEIN

Pea protein powder is a supplement made by extracting protein from yellow peas. It's typically used to increase the protein content of smoothies. Pea protein contains all nine essential amino acids that your body cannot create and must get from food. Other great plant powder protein sources you can use in the recipes in this book are rice, hemp, quinoa, and chia.

REISHI

The reishi mushroom was first discovered by Chinese healers more than 2,000 years ago in the Changbai Mountains. Within the mushroom, there are several molecules, including triterpenoids, polysaccharides, and peptidoglycans, that may be responsible for its health effects. Reishi mushroom extract has been shown to encourage the body to relax, making it easier to fall asleep and improving the quality of sleep.

SHATAVARI

Native to India, shatavari is an adaptogen that supports hormone health. Called the "queen of herbs," it supports fertility and hormone health. Ayurveda uses shatavari to treat conditions related to hormone imbalance such as polycystic ovarian syndrome (PCOS) and infertility and to reduce symptoms of menopause. Shatavari powder comes from the roots of the *Asparagus racemosus* plant—yes, it's related to the asparagus!

SPIRULINA

Spirulina is an organism that grows in both fresh and saltwater. It's a type of cyanobacteria, a family of single-celled microbes that appeared on Earth 3.5 billion years ago and are often referred to as "blue-green algae." It's particularly recognizable for its spiral shape. Spirulina is about 60 percent protein and is also a good source of B vitamins, copper, and iron; decent amounts of magnesium, potassium, and manganese; and small amounts of almost every other nutrient that you need. Spirulina was consumed by the ancient Aztecs but became popular again when NASA proposed that it could be grown in space for use by astronauts.

TOCOS

Tocos is derived from the bran of organically grown brown rice. It's known as a super-rich source of fat-soluble vitamin E, which is exceptional for connective tissue and skin. It may also protect the skin from air pollution and other chemical irritants. You can even take rice bran solubles as a nutritional supplement, sometimes called "tocos" because of their high content of tocopherols (vitamin E).

TULSI

Tulsi is an adaptogen that helps calm your nervous system and reduce stress. It's an aromatic shrub in the basil family that is thought to have originated in north-central India. Also called "holy basil" the plant is widely used in Ayurvedic and folk medicine, often as an herbal tea for a variety of ailments. It contains vitamins A and C, calcium, zinc, iron, and chlorophyll and is known to support mood and sleep and buffer stress.

TURMERIC

Analysis of pots discovered near New Delhi has uncovered residue from turmeric that dates back as early as 2500 BCE. It was around 500 BCE that turmeric emerged as an important part of Ayurvedic medicine. Many high-quality studies show that turmeric has major benefits for your body and brain. Many of these benefits come from its main active ingredient, curcumin. Curcumin is a potent antioxidant that can neutralize free radicals because of its chemical structure. Curcumin boosts levels of the brain hormone BDNF, which increases the growth of new neurons and may help fight various degenerative processes in your brain. Curcumin also has beneficial effects on several factors known to play a role in heart disease. Plus, it's an anti-inflammatory agent and antioxidant.

WHEATGRASS

Wheatgrass can be traced back in history over 5,000 years to ancient Egypt and perhaps even early Mesopotamian civilizations. It is purported that ancient Egyptians considered the young leafy blades of wheat sacred and prized them for their positive effect on health and vitality. Wheatgrass contains iron, calcium, magnesium, phytonutrients, 17 amino acids, and vitamins A, C, E, K, and B complex. Like all green plants, wheatgrass also contains chlorophyll, a type of green-plant pigment associated with many health benefits.

You can find more detail on each one of these throughout the recipes in the book; for a quick glance at what they are, where they most commonly come from, and what they do for us and why, check out the handy chart on page 22 you can refer back to as you start to play with adding them to your day. We also include suggested serving size, and taste and color, so that you have an idea of what you're looking for and how to combine them during cooking.

All superfoods come from plants—whether mushrooms, fruits, algae, seeds, roots, or grasses. Some can be labeled adaptogens, which are particularly known to work with your body to create more balance and reduce stress.

You'll see that we've noted what they're especially good for—skin health, stress management, mood boost, healthy fats, detox and immunity, energy, plant protein, hormone health, and fighting inflammation. We've labeled recipes with these categories throughout the book so that if you're particularly concerned about getting better immunity, for example, you can go right to those recipes. See below for a list of our top 10 superfoods to help you get going if you're overwhelmed or unsure where to start. Keep in mind, though, that in most recipes the superfoods are optional so you can still enjoy the dishes even if you don't have all the superfoods at home!

GETTING STARTING WITH THE TOP 10 SUPERFOODS

Don't feel like you have to run out to by all 25 superfoods at once. If you want an easy way to get started, here is the list of the top 10 most used superfoods that offer you good variety when starting out.

1. Açaí
2. Cacao
3. Wheatgrass
4. Turmeric
5. Reishi
6. Pea Protein
7. Chia Seeds
8. Ginger
9. Ashwagandha
10. Maca

SUPERFOOD POWDER	WHAT IT IS	COUNTRIES GROWN	BENEFIT
AÇAÍ BERRY	Berry	Brazil	Skin health
ACEROLA	Cherry	Brazil, Mexico	Immunity
ASHWAGANDHA	Root	India, Asia, Africa	Stress management
BAOBAB	Fruit	Africa	Immunity
CACAO	Bean	South America	Mood booster
CHAGA	Mushroom	China, Northern Europe, Canada	Immunity
CHIA SEEDS	Small seeds	South America	Healthy fats
CHLORELLA	Algae	Germany, Japan, Taiwan	Detoxing
FLAXSEEDS	Seeds	Canada, United States, India, China	Healthy fats
GINGER	Root	India, China, Indonesia	Immunity
GUARANA	Seeds	Brazil, South America	Energy
HEMP PROTEIN	Protein from hemp plant	Canada, United States, Europe	Plant protein
KELP	Seaweed	Oceans	Energy
MACA	Root	Peru	Hormone health
MAQUI	Berry	Chile, Argentina	Skin health
MATCHA	Plant leaves	Japan	Energy
MORINGA	Tree leaves	India, Africa	Energy
PEA PROTEIN	Pea	Belgium, Canada, China	Plant protein
REISHI	Mushroom	China, Southern Europe	Stress management
SHATAVARI	Root	India, Sri Lanka	Hormone health
SPIRULINA	Algae	Many countries, including Chile, Germany, China	Detoxing
TOCOS	Rice bran solubles	Asia	Skin health
TULSI	Herb	India	Stress management
TURMERIC	Root	India	Anti-inflammatory
WHEATGRASS	Young grass	United States, Germany, New Zealand	Detoxing

	SERVING SIZE	TASTE	COLOR	COMBINES WELL WITH . . .
	1 teaspoon	Tart berry	Dark purple	Maqui, acerola, tocos, maca, pea protein
	1 teaspoon	Sour cherry	Light orange	Baobab, açaí, maqui
	½ teaspoon	Bitter	White	Cacao, turmeric, shatavari, tocos
	1 teaspoon	Fresh, sour lemon-ish	Light yellow	Acerola, ginger, açaí, maqui, wheatgrass, chlorella
	2 teaspoons	Bitter chocolate	Dark brown	Shatavari, reishi, pea protein, maca, chaga
	½ teaspoon	Bitter mushroom	Dark brown	Reishi, cacao, maca, guarana
	2 tablespoons	No taste	Gray, white	Anything
	1 teaspoon	Green	Bright green	Baobab, spirulina, wheatgrass, moringa
	1 teaspoon	Nutty	Brown	Anything
	½ teaspoon	Spicy	Light yellow	Turmeric, tulsi, matcha, baoabab, acerola
	½ teaspoon	Nutty, bitter	Dark brown	Açaí, maqui, chaga, reishi, cacao
	2 tbsp	Green, earthy	Green	Spirulina, chlorella, kelp
	½ teaspoon	Fishy	Dark green	Spirulina, chlorella, hemp protein
	½ teaspoon	Bitter, slightly sweet	White, light yellow	Açaí, maqui, tocos, pea protein, cacao, shatavari
	1 teaspoon	Bitter berry	Dark purple	Açaí, acerola, baobab, tocos, pea protein
	½ teaspoon	Green tea	Bright green	Turmeric, ginger, moringa, wheatgrass, cacao
	1 teaspoon	Green, a little like tea	Green	Baobab, spirulina, chlorella, wheatgrass, tulsi
	2 tablespoons	Neutral, pea taste	Cream, off white	Anything
	½ teaspoon	Bitter mushroom	Dark brown	Cacao, chaga, guarana, maca
	½ teaspoon	Bitter	Creamy, off-white	Maca, ashwagandha, tocos, açaí, cacao
	½ teaspoon	Very green	Dark green	Baobab, chlorella, moringa, wheatgrass
	2 teaspoons	Slightly sweet, neutral	Creamy, white	Açaí, maqui, pea protein, shatavari, maca, ashwagandha
	½ teaspoon	Bitter, slightly sweet	Green	Turmeric, ginger, moringa
	½ teaspoon	Spicy	Bright orange	Ginger, ashwagandha, cinnamon
	1 teaspoon	Slightly sweet, grassy	Green	Baobab, spirulina, chlorella, moringa

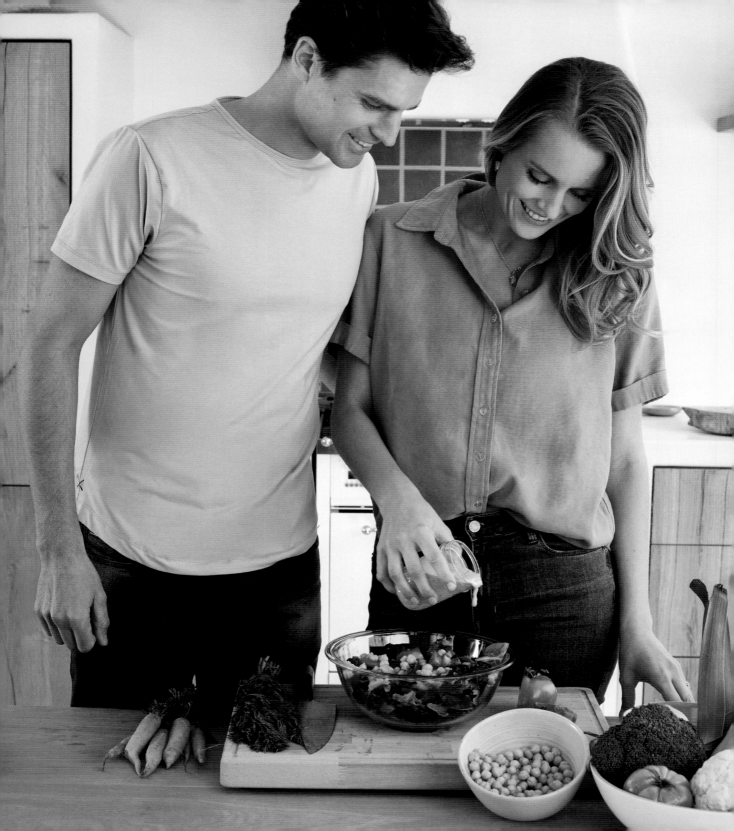

YOUR SUPER LIFE KITCHEN

Now that you know about the incredible benefits of superfoods and plant-based eating, let's get ready to cook! The first step in transitioning to this plant-powered lifestyle is preparing your kitchen and pantry by stocking up on all of the essentials you need—don't worry, we make this simple for you, too.

Here is a list of pantry items you'll want to have stocked, along with grocery lists for the recipes in this book. You may have some of these on hand already. But if not, don't stress. The next time you go to the grocery store, stock up on the dry ingredients, the canned and jarred items, and the condiments and spices so that you always have them ready to go. Pick up fresh fruits and veggies during your weekly grocery haul, or, even better, from a farmers market if they're in season.

You can be flexible when it comes to your produce: What is in season? What is easily available near you? The recipes are designed with a mix of fruits and veggies so that you get a variety of nutrients in your diet. Let this list inspire you and spark ideas about what fruits and veggies you can add to your weekly rotation. These are all the ingredients we used to make the recipes in this book.

Grocery List

FRESH FRUITS

Apple
Banana
Raspberries
Blueberries
Strawberries

Lemon
Lime
Melon
Orange
Passion fruit

Peach
Mango
Nectarine
Apricot

FRESH VEGETABLES

Avocado
Basil
Beet
Bell pepper, red or yellow
Broccoli
Carrots
Celery
Cilantro
Corn

Cucumber
Eggplant
Garlic
Ginger root
Green peas
Kale leaves
Lettuce
Leek
Mint

Mushrooms
Onions
Potatoes
Scallions
Spinach
Sprouts
Tomatoes
Turmeric root
Zucchini

FROZEN FOODS

Blueberries
Corn
Edamame beans

Green peas
Mango
Raspberries

Spinach
Strawberries

PANTRY STAPLES

Almonds
Almond butter
Almond flour
Almond milk
Bread, gluten-free
Cashews
Cashew butter
Coconut milk
Coconut, shredded
Coconut sugar
Coconut water
Corn taco shells
Dates

Flaxseed crackers
Lentils, red
Hazelnut butter
Herbal teas
Noodles
Oats, quick
Oat milk
Peanut butter
Pecans
Pasta, gluten-free
Pistachios
Popcorn kernels
Pumpkin seeds

Quinoa
Raisins
Rice, brown
Rice cakes
Sesame seeds
Sunflower seeds
Tahini
Tempeh
Tofu
Walnuts
Wraps, gluten-free
Vegetable broth powder
Yogurt, plant-based

CANNED AND JARRED

Artichokes
Black beans
Capers
Chickpeas

Jackfruit
Kidney beans
Olives
Sun-dried tomatoes

Tomato paste and sauce
White beans, cannellini or navy

CONDIMENTS

Apple vinegar
Balsamic vinegar
Coconut aminos
Coconut oil

Maple syrup
Mustard, whole grain
Olive oil
Sesame oil

Soy sauce
Sriracha sauce
Tamari sauce
Vanilla extract

SPICES

Black pepper
Chili powder
Cinnamon powder
Cumin powder

Curry powder
Dill
Garlic powder
Italian herbs

Nori flakes
Nutritional yeast
Onion powder
Sea salt

SUPERFOODS

Superfoods (see table, page 22) or Your Super mixes (see page 281)

SUPERFOOD SUCCESS STORY

DANIELLE

I started with the Detox Bundle with superfoods like turmeric, ginger, moringa, chlorella, acerola, and spirulina. I was in my mid-40s and perimenopausal with a general lack of energy. I felt the weight of eating poorly for a few years and working in a restaurant nearly 24/7. I can tell you the detox made me feel like myself again! I felt good, whole, energetic . . . and to my surprise, I smelled better! The usual body odor that was my "normal" was gone. Since the detox, I've continued using most of your powders every single day in my morning smoothie. I've been exposed to COVID and other viruses and haven't been sick yet! I attribute that to Your Super powders helping me build up a strong immune system!

Kitchen Tools

This is a short list—simply because you don't need a lot. Some of the basics, especially a really good blender, a ceramic-coated cooking pan, and some good knives, make all the difference in the world. You'll see that we recommend wooden or bamboo cutting boards and utensils over plastic. If you cut–cut–cut every day on the same plastic board, at some point small pieces of plastic might get into your food, and we want to avoid that. We want to avoid getting plastics into our food, whether it's from a plastic cutting board or the utensils used in a hot stir-fry pan. That damage from everyday use allows toxins to enter your food. Remember, plastic utensils are heat-resistant to 400 degrees, not heatproof. They will melt with extended contact with a hot pan.

BASICS

- **HIGH-SPEED BLENDER:** Smoothies, power balls, soups, you name it, you will use your blender every day. Invest a little bit of extra money to get a high-speed version—we love the Vitamix blender but there are many other good options.
- **CERAMIC-COATED PANS:** Stock up on three basic versions: a pan, a wok, and a pot. I often buy mine at TJ Maxx. The amazing thing about ceramic-coated pans is that you can cut down on the amount of oil in your cooking; if you stir-fry with just a little water, your food won't burn and stick to the pan.
- **SHARP KNIVES:** A good, sharp chef's knife makes veggie prep so much easier!
- **CUTTING BOARD:** Wooden or bamboo (instead of plastic).
- **FROTHER:** Great for making quick lattes. A handheld stick is all you need.
- **THINGS YOU PROBABLY ALREADY HAVE:** A strainer, can opener, oven rack, and chlorine-free parchment paper, and wooden or bamboo utensils for stir-frying (instead of plastic).

OPTIONAL

- **SLOW JUICER:** Perfect for making delicious juices. However, these can be a hassle to clean so I often opt to simply make smoothies.
- **STACKABLE SPROUT KIT:** You can usually find cheap sprouting kits on Amazon if you want to try growing your own sprouts at home. Mung bean sprouts are especially easy and super delicious.

Should I Buy Organic?

We try to eat mostly organic produce and food products because:

- Organic food contains fewer pesticides, fewer additives and preservatives, and no GMO ingredients (meaning the crops have not been genetically modified).
- Organically produced crops (cereals, fruit, and vegetables) have been found to have up to 68 percent more antioxidants than nonorganic, and organic fruit and veggies contain lower concentrations of pesticides and the toxic heavy metal cadmium.[1]
- Organic farming is better for the planet as it doesn't use artificial fertilizers, which results in healthier soils that store more carbon.

If it's not possible to buy everything organic, be sure to clean your fruit and veggies well.

1. Fill a large bowl with 4 parts water to 1 part plain white vinegar.
2. Soak the fruits or vegetables in the mixture for 20 minutes.
3. Rinse the fruits or vegetables well with water.

The Dirty Dozen and Clean 15 guidelines can help you prioritize when to buy organic and when conventional is okay. Certain conventionally grown fruits and vegetables contain more pesticides than others, so prioritize buying those organic. Produce on the clean list has a lower pesticide residue than produce on the dirty list. For instance, strawberries have been on top of the dirty list for years—22 different pesticide residues have been found there!

CLEAN

Avocado, sweet corn, pineapple, onion, papaya, sweet peas, asparagus, cabbage, kiwi, mushrooms, honeydew melon, cantaloupe, mangoes, sweet potatoes, watermelon

DIRTY

Strawberries, spinach, kale, collard greens, mustard greens, nectarines, apples, grapes, cherries, peaches, pears, bell and hot peppers, celery, tomatoes

STEPHANIE

I used to suffer from migraines more days in a month than I didn't. I'd tried all avenues of medication with temporary or no results, and I was running out of options. After researching diet changes and their potential for migraine relief, I found the Your Super detox. During my first detox I experienced migraine-free days for the first time in weeks. My energy was way up too! I have continued to do occasional detoxes, with superfoods like ginger, maca, açaí, chia seeds, ashwagandha, tocos, and turmeric as well as using the mixes in my everyday diet. I particularly enjoy Super Green, Golden Mellow, Plant Collagen, and Plant Protein. Afterward, I have noticed a drastic change in the frequency and severity of migraines. I also crave fewer sweets, salty foods, and red meats. Overall the experience has made me more aware of the foods and additives that trigger migraines, has given me more energy, and is a good complement to a healthier lifestyle.

A WORD ON PLANT-BASED ALTERNATIVES

We love plant-based alternatives like vegan ice cream and cheese, but some of them are highly processed foods that we don't want to eat every day. Vegan pizza and burgers taste amazing and we are so happy they exist, but while we enjoy them occasionally, we don't recommend making them a daily habit. Instead, focus on eating plants in their natural, whole-food form. Read ingredient labels when you buy packaged foods.

A WORD ON SUGAR, SWEETENERS, SALT, AND OILS

If you want something sweet, go for whole foods like fruits, maple syrup, and dates. We don't like highly processed sweeteners, like white or brown sugar, or even stevia and xylitol. The problem with them—even the calorie-free options—is that your brain still recognizes them as something sweet, and insulin spikes to process the sugar that is not there. Normally the hormone insulin helps move the glucose available from the foods you eat from your bloodstream and into your cells, which use it for fuel at a later point. If there is no glucose there but your insulin spikes, you can be hungrier *after* eating.

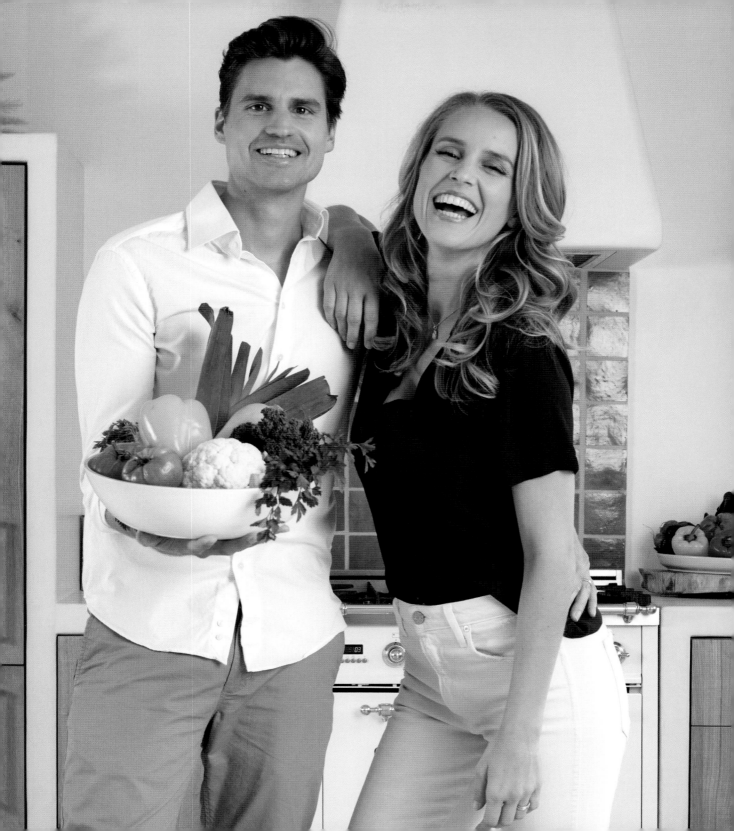

One thing you should never shy away from is fruit—we love fruit! People are afraid of fruit because of its sugar content, and we need to change that fear. Fruit has many vitamins, minerals, antioxidants, phytonutrients, and fiber that your body needs to be healthy. There is a difference between natural and processed sugar. The sugar in a banana is not the same as white sugar or high-fructose corn syrup. Think of it this way: If it grows naturally and you're eating it in its natural form, it can't be that bad for you.

You will often find our recipes call for "salt and pepper to taste." Black pepper is great to use as desired, because it actually supports and increases your nutrient absorption. For salt, we recommend you use sea salt or Himalayan pink salt and use it sparingly. Many of us eat way too much salt, and more than we realize: It's heavily added to processed foods and in restaurants and takeout. When you start reducing your salt intake, you will notice that your taste buds start to change and adapt to lower levels. Before long, you'll be eating in a restaurant and wondering why things taste so salty.

While healthy fats from whole foods like avocado, nuts, coconut, seeds (like chia or sesame seeds), and nut and seed butters are great for your health, try to reduce processed oils like olive oil, sunflower oil, and coconut oil. They're okay in small amounts, but they're not something that should be consumed in large amounts. If you use oil, we recommend organic, cold-pressed oils like olive oil and coconut oil. As you will see, we use minimal oil in our recipes, and prefer to cook or stir-fry with water, which works well in ceramic-coated cookware.

LET YOUR BODY REST

One tip you might want to try is to pause between your last meal of the day and your first meal after waking. We try not to have any food or drink (other than water) for 10 to 12 hours between the last meal and breakfast. It's a lot of work for your body to digest and process food. This mini fast gives your body time to do something other than digesting food: to cleanse, recover, and reset. It's a small tip that can make a difference to your health.

Supplements

You get an abundance of nutrients from whole fruits, vegetables, seeds, legumes, and grains in the plant kingdom, but supplementing with some nutrients can be helpful. You also might want to consider having your blood levels tested once a year. Supplement with:

- **VITAMIN B$_{12}$:** This is a key vitamin to supplement if you're fully plant-based, but it's important even if you don't eat a plant-based diet. B$_{12}$ comes from soil bacteria, and the soil is less nutrient-rich today than it was generations ago, so there's less and less B$_{12}$ in the soil. B$_{12}$ is important for many body functions. Aim for at least 2.4 micrograms per day.
- **VITAMIN D$_3$:** We used to get vitamin D through our skin from sun exposure, but most people today are deficient in vitamin D thanks to our modern lifestyles. Recommendations range from 400 IU up to the thousands. We like to follow the recommendation of leading vegan researcher and physician Michael Greger, MD, who advises a supplement of 2,000 IU per day. D$_3$ is often derived from animal sources, so look for a vegan source, usually mushrooms.
- **DHA & EPA:** These omega-3 fatty acids come from algae. We go straight to the source, which is the algae that the fish eat. Aim for 300 mg DHA, 100 to 200 mg EPA.

When sourcing supplements, be mindful of where these vitamins or minerals come from. Ninety percent of supplements are synthetically derived. You want to look for supplements that are derived from real whole foods.

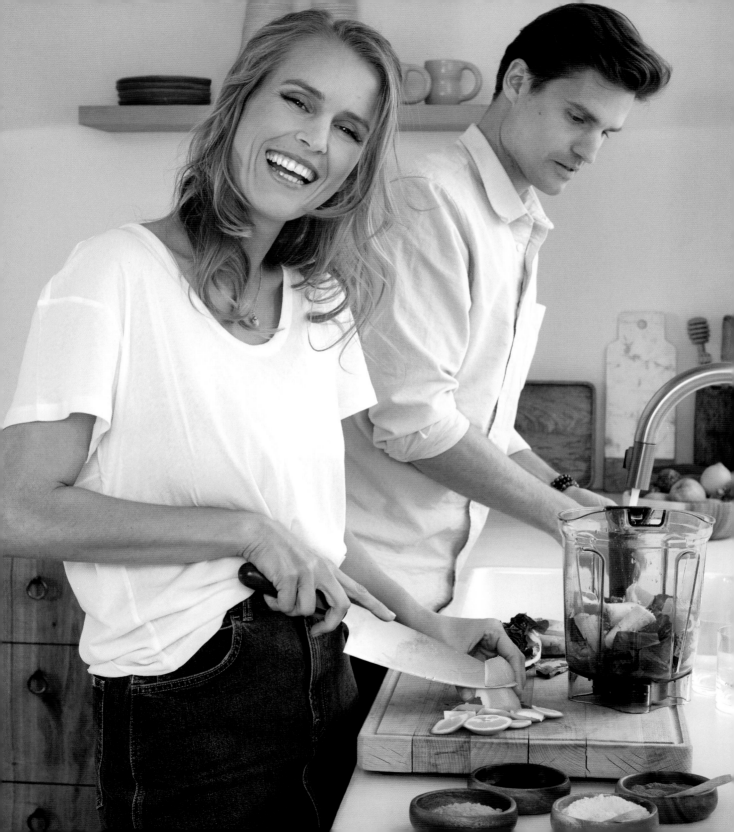

YOUR WEEKLY MEAL PLANS

We want this book to work for you, so feel free to skip this section if you're more of a free-flow kind of person who prefers not to plan ahead. You'll use the general shopping lists to help you start building your pantry staples and then make decisions at the grocery store based on what you're in the mood to eat, choosing from any recipe in this book. The "How To" sections in each chapter will totally be your jam (see list on page xvii).

But if you're the type of person who loves to make a list and plan your meals once a week, or if you're just beginning to change your diet and want some additional structure and help planning, we created three weekly meal plans with accompanying grocery lists. Some people find a weekly plan easier than deciding what to eat in the moment, especially when you might be hungry, tired, or stressed—and don't have the right ingredients on hand.

The first plan is an Everyday Health plan, which is the perfect place to start if you simply want to focus on eating a week of plant-based foods and incorporate superfoods. The second weekly meal plan focuses on Skin and Hormone Health, and the third on Detox, Immunity, and Anti-inflammatory benefits. You will also find an empty weekly meal plan and grocery list, which you can fill out by yourself with your favorite recipes to plan your week.

Remember: This is not a diet and we don't want you to deprive yourself. You should not feel hungry when following these meal plans. Make sure to drink lots of water so you stay hydrated. All recipes are easily doubled if you need to make the serving sizes larger. Trust your body and learn to eat when you are hungry and stop eating when you are full. We include three optional snacks with each daily plan. Maybe you will feel satisfied with the three main meals, or maybe you'll want something extra. It's up to you.

These recipes offer a lot of options for ingredients. In the grocery lists below, an * indicates an ingredient that is optional in the recipes in that meal plan, such as for toppings, garnishes, or superfood ingredients. You can also download and print plans and grocery lists online at **kristelandmichael.com**.

EVERYDAY HEALTH MEAL PLAN

	MONDAY	TUESDAY	WEDNESDAY	THURSDAY	FRIDAY	SATURDAY	SUNDAY
BREAKFAST	Protein Berry Smoothie 67	Creamy Turmeric Oats 73	Fruity Green Smoothie 79	Berry Oats Overnight 59	Fruity Green Smoothie 79	Chocolate Protein Smoothie 70	Tofu Veggie Scramble 89
SNACK	Matcha Latte 105	Chocolate-Dipped Strawberries 121	Chocolate-Dipped Strawberries 121	Super Apple Slices 119	Chagachino 107	Carrot Cake Balls 117	Carrot Cake Balls 117
LUNCH	Easy Green Salad 137	Easy Green Salad 137	Mexican-Style Bowl 149	Mexican-Style Bowl 149	Italian-Inspired Antipasto Salad 143	Thai-Inspired Peanut Salad 163	Thai-Inspired Peanut Salad 163
SNACK	Superfood Popcorn (Berries) 198	Berrylicious Milkshake 183	Superfood Popcorn (Berries) 198	Superfood Popcorn (Berries) 198	Roasted Chickpeas 194	Roasted Chickpeas 194	Roasted Chickpeas 194
DINNER	Eggplant Pasta 209	Eggplant Pasta 209	Easy Green Stir-Fry 207	Mexican-Inspired Chili Bowl 220	Mexican-Inspired Chili Bowl 220	Veggie Melanzane 231	Veggie Melanzane 231
DESSERT	Calming Chocolate Latte 253	Creamy Chocolate Dates 263	Relaxing Turmeric Latte 251	Creamy Chocolate Dates 263	Tropical Ice Cream 257	Banana Split Bowl 265	Healthy Chocolate Mousse 259

Everyday Health Grocery List

FRESH FRUITS

Apple, 1

Banana, 6

Lemon, 2

Limes, 3

Orange, 2

Raspberries, ½ cup

Strawberries, 2 cups

FRESH VEGETABLES

Avocados, 3

Basil, 1 bunch

Bell peppers, red, 3

Carrots, 3

Cilantro, 1 bunch

Cucumbers, 2

Eggplants, 2

Garlic cloves, 2

Kale, 5 leaves

Mushrooms, button, 2 cups

Mushrooms, portobellos, 2

Onions, red, 1

Onions, white, 4

Potatoes, sweet, 2 cups

Romaine lettuce, 2 heads

Scallions, 11

Spinach, fresh, 6 cups

*Sprouts, alfalfa or broccoli

Tomato, 10

Zucchini, 3

FROZEN FOODS

*Berries, mixed, ½ cup

Blueberries, 1⅓ cups

Cauliflower, ½ cup

Corn, 3 cups

Edamame beans, 2 cups

Mango, 1 cup

Peas, 1 cup

Strawberries, 1 cup

PANTRY STAPLES

Almonds, ¼ cup

Almond butter, ¾ cup

Almond milk, 2½ cups

Artichokes, 1 can

Beans, black, 1 can

Beans, chickpeas, 2 cans

Beans kidney, 1 can

Beans, white, 2 cans

Capers, 4 tablespoons

Cashews, 2 cups

Coconut milk, 2 cans

*Coconut, shredded, ¼ cup

Dates, 11

*Flaxseed crackers, 1 cup

Hazelnut butter, 1 tablespoon

Oats, quick, 2 cups

Oat milk, 1 cup

Olives, ¼ cup

Pasta, gluten-free, 12 ounces

Peanut butter, 4¼ cups

Plant milk, oat or almond, 2½ quarts

Popcorn kernels, ¼ cup

Pumpkin seeds, 4 tablespoons

Raisins, 1¼ cups

Rice, brown, 2 cups

Tomato paste, 1 cup

Tomato sauce, 4 cups

Tofu, firm, 12 ounces

Tahini, ½ cup

Yogurt, almond or soy, 1 cup

CONDIMENTS

Balsamic vinegar

Coconut oil

Maple syrup

Nutritional yeast

Sriracha sauce

Tamari sauce

*Vanilla extract

SPICES

Black pepper

Cinnamon powder

Chili powder

Cumin powder

Curry powder

Garlic powder

Italian herbs

Nutritional yeast

Oregano

Sea salt

SUPERFOODS

Açaí powder

*Acerola powder

*Ashwagandha powder

*Baobab powder

Cacao powder

Cacao nibs

Chaga powder

Chia seeds

*Chlorella powder

Flaxseeds

Ginger powder

*Guarana powder

*Hemp protein powder

*Maca powder

*Maqui powder

Matcha powder

*Moringa powder

Pea protein powder

*Reishi powder

*Spirulina powder

*Tocos powder

*Tulsi powder

Turmeric powder

Wheatgrass powder

SKIN AND HORMONE HEALTH MEAL PLAN

	MONDAY	TUESDAY	WEDNESDAY	THURSDAY	FRIDAY	SATURDAY	SUNDAY
BREAKFAST	Berry Hormone Smoothie 83	Berry Hormone Smoothie 83	Protein Berry Smoothie 67	Protein Berry Smoothie 67	Easy Açaí Bowl 61	Easy Açaí Bowl 61	Berry Oats Overnight 59
SNACK	Happy Hormones Latte 103	Berry Balls 113	Happy Hormones Latte 103	Berry Balls 113	Happy Hormones Latte 103	Berry Balls 113	Berry Balls 113
LUNCH	Mexican-Style Bowl 149	Mexican-Style Bowl 149	Easy Green Salad 137	Easy Green Salad 137	Creamy Tomato Soup 159	Creamy Tomato Soup 159	Tomato Tofu Platter 139
SNACK	Berrylicious Milkshake 183	Energizing Berry Water 179	Energizing Berry Watter 179	Berrylicious Milkshake 183	Kidney Bean Hummus 187	Kidney Bean Hummus 187	Kidney Bean Hummus 187
DINNER	Roasted Rainbow Veggies 219	Roasted Rainbow Veggies 219	Roasted Rainbow Veggies 219	Lentil Stew 226	Lentil Stew 226	Stir-Fry Noodles 230	Stir-Fry Noodles 230
DESSERT	Creamy Chocolate Dates 263	Relaxing Turmeric Latte 251	Relaxing Turmeric Latte 251	Creamy Chocolate Dates 263	Homemade Immunity Tea 255	Happy Brownies 277	Happy Brownies 277

Skin and Hormone Health Grocery List

FRESH FRUITS

Banana, 5

*Berries, mixed, 1 cup

Lemon, 2

Lime, 2

FRESH VEGETABLES

Avocado, 11

Basil, 1 bunch

Beet, 1

Bell pepper, red, 4

Broccoli, 1 cup

Button mushrooms, 3 cups

Carrots, 4

Cilantro, 1 bunch

Cucumber, 1

Garlic cloves, 13

Ginger root, 2 inches

Leek, 1

Mint, 1 bunch

Romaine lettuce, 2 heads

Onions, white, 4

Potatoes, 6

Potatoes, sweet, 2 cups

Scallions, 10

Spinach, 1 cup

Tomatoes, 10

Turmeric root, 1 inch

Zucchini, 1

FROZEN FOODS

Blueberries, 3⅓ cups

Cauliflower, ½ cup

Corn, 1 cup

Raspberries, 2½ cups

Strawberries, 2 cups

PANTRY STAPLES

Almonds, ¾ cup

Almond butter, ½ cup

Almond flour, 1 cup

Almond milk, ¾ cup

Beans, black, 1 can

Beans, chickpeas, 1 can

Beans kidney, 1 can

Beans, white, 1 can

Capers, 4 tablespoons

Cashews, ¾ cup

Coconut milk, 2 cups

Coconut, shredded, 2 tablespoons

Dates, 4 cups

*Flaxseed crackers, 1 cup

Lentils, red, 1½ cups

Noodles, rice or buckwheat, 8 ounces

Oats, quick, 2 cups

Oat milk, 1 cup

Plant milk, oat or almond, 2½ quarts

Pumpkin seeds, ¼ cup

Raisins, 2 tablespoons

*Sesame seeds, ¼ cup

Tahini, ¾ cup

Tomato paste, ⅓ cup

Tofu, firm, 12 ounces

Tahini, 4 tablespoons

*Vegetable broth powder, ¼ cup

Yogurt, almond or soy, 1½ cups

CONDIMENTS

Balsamic vinegar

Coconut oil

Maple syrup

Nutritional yeast

*Olive oil

Sriracha sauce

Tamari sauce

*Vanilla extract

SPICES

Black pepper

Cinnamon powder

Chili powder

Cumin powder

Garlic powder

Italian herbs

Sea salt

SUPERFOODS

Açaí powder

*Acerola powder

*Baobab powder

Cacao nibs

Cacao powder

Chia seeds

*Guarana powder

*Hemp protein powder

Maca powder

*Maqui powder

*Moringa powder

Pea protein powder

*Reishi powder

Spirulina powder

*Tocos powder

*Tulsi powder

Turmeric powder

DETOX, IMMUNITY, AND ANTI-INFLAMMATORY MEAL PLAN

	MONDAY	TUESDAY	WEDNESDAY	THURSDAY	FRIDAY	SATURDAY	SUNDAY
BREAKFAST	Fruity Green Smoothie 79	Fruity Green Smoothie 79	All Green Smoothie 81	All Green Smoothie 81	Classic Green Smoothie 65	Classic Green Smoothie 65	Tropical Yellow Smoothie Bowl 77
SNACK	Super Apple Slices 119	Protein Oat Cookies 123	Super Apple Slices 119	Protein Oat Cookies 123	Green Super Balls 109	Green Super Balls 109	Green Super Balls 109
LUNCH	Potato Dill Salad 141	Potato Dill Salad 141	Zucchini Pasta Salad 157	Healthy Sprout Salad 154	Healthy Sprout Salad 154	Green Soup 147	Green Soup 147
SNACK	Detox Water 178	Baobab Lemonade 175	Sparkling Turmeric Refresher 177	Great Northern Bean Hummus 189	Great Northern Bean Hummus 189	Roasted Nuts 193	Roasted Nuts 193
DINNER	Easy Green Stir-Fry 207	Easy Green Stir-Fry 207	Plant Power Bowl 225	Plant Power Bowl 225	Easy Pumpkin Curry 217	Easy Pumpkin Curry 217	Easy Pumpkin Curry 217
DESSERT	Homemade Immunity Tea 255	Turmeric Bounty Balls 275	Relaxing Turmeric Latte 251	Turmeric Bounty Balls 275	Relaxing Turmeric Latte 251	Turmeric Bounty Balls 275	Homemade Immunity Tea 255

Detox, Immunity, and Anti-inflammatory Grocery List

FRESH FRUITS

Apples, 2

Bananas, 5

Lemons, 3

Limes, 2

Oranges, 3

FRESH VEGETABLES

Avocado 4½

Basil, 1 bunch

Bell pepper, red, 1

Broccoli, 2 heads

Carrots, 2

*Cilantro, 1 bunch

Cucumbers, 3

Dill, 1 bunch

Ginger root, 5½ inches

Kale, 3 cups

Mung bean sprouts, 2 cups

Onions, 3

Parsley, 1 bunch

Potatoes, 4

Potatoes, purple sweet, 2

Pumpkin or butternut squash, 1

Romaine lettuce, 1 head

Scallions, 1

Sprouts, alfalfa or broccoli, 4 cups

Salad greens, mixed, 6 cups

Spinach, 3 cups

Tomatoes, 1

Turmeric root, 1 inch

Zucchini, 3

FROZEN FOODS

Edamame beans, 1 cup

Mango, 1 cup

Peas, 1 cup

Pineapple, ½ cup

Spinach, 2 cups

PANTRY STAPLES

Almonds, 1 cup

Almond butter, ½ cup

Dates, pitted, 1 cup

Beans, chickpeas, 1 can

Beans kidney, 1 can

Beans, white, 1 can

Cashews, 1¼ cup

Coconut milk, 2 cans

Coconut water, 1½ cups

*Coconut, shredded, ¼ cup

Dates, 11

*Flaxseed crackers, 4 cups

Oats, quick, 2 cups

Oat milk, ½ cup

*Olives, kalamata, ½ cup

Peanut butter, ¼ cup

Plant milk, oat or almond, 3 cups

Raisins, ⅓ cup

Rice, brown, 4 cups

Sauerkraut, ½ cup

Sparkling water, 1½ cups

*Sunflower seeds, ⅛ cup

Sun-dried tomatoes, 1 jar

Tahini, ¾ cup

Tofu, firm, 24 ounces

CONDIMENTS

Coconut oil

Maple syrup

Mustard, whole grain

Tamari sauce

SPICES

Black pepper

Cinnamon powder

Chili powder

Curry powder

Dill

Garlic powder

Italian herbs

*Nori or kelp flakes

Sea salt

SUPERFOODS

Açaí powder

*Acerola powder

*Ashwagandha powder

Baobab powder

*Chlorella powder

Ginger powder

*Hemp protein powder

*Moringa powder

Pea protein powder

*Spirulina powder

*Tocos powder

*Tulsi powder

Turmeric powder

Wheatgrass powder

YOUR WEEKLY MEAL PLAN

Found your favorite recipes? Write out your week's plan of what you plan on eating and making. You can always double a recipe so that you can enjoy leftovers tomorrow and save time in the kitchen.

	MONDAY	TUESDAY	WEDNESDAY	THURSDAY	FRIDAY	SATURDAY	SUNDAY
BREAKFAST							
SNACK							
LUNCH							
SNACK							
DINNER							
DESSERT							
GROCERY LIST							

GO AT YOUR PACE

If these plans make you feel overwhelmed and going 100 percent plant-based right now feels like too big of a stretch . . . then don't do it! The goal is to take steps in the right direction; you don't have to overhaul your entire lifestyle in one day. Maybe you want to start by eating one plant-based meal a day. Or maybe you feel ready to eat plant-based five days a week, and then let it go on the weekends. Some choose to target one food group or animal product at a time.

No matter how you choose to start, as you add more healthy, plant-based food to your lifestyle, you'll begin to slowly crowd out and cut back on unhealthy foods. Over time your cravings will dissipate and disappear; this happens without restricting, you just followed your taste buds as they changed. Celebrate every win and slowly start noticing the difference in how you feel. Remember there is no right or wrong way—you got this!

CHART THE CHANGES

At the end of a week of plant-based eating and incorporating superfoods, use the chart on the next page to track how you are feeling. Many people experience the benefits of more energy, feeling lighter, less bloated, and/or having better skin very quickly. Note that some people experience detox symptoms like headaches or congestion in the first 2 to 4 days after transitioning their diets, which is normal and will go away. Reflecting helps to create awareness of how good you are feeling when you eat this way, and how you feel day to day. Feeling good is what it's all about.

SELF CHECK-IN CHART

I AM FEELING . . .

CHECK ALL THAT APPLY	☐ Happy	☐ Excited	☐ Sad	☐ Anxious	☐ Hungry
	☐ Tired	☐ Lonely	☐ Bored	☐ Light	☐ Energetic
	☐ Hopeful	☐ Defeated	☐ Empowered	☐ Confident	☐ Grateful

I AM PROUD OF . . .

MY ENERGY LEVELS ARE . . .

☐ 1	☐ 2	☐ 3	☐ 4	☐ 5

MY DIGESTION THIS WEEK

☐ Every Day	☐ Every Other Day	☐ Irregular & Struggling

NEXT WEEK I WANT TO CONTINUE . . .

WHAT I LEARNED I CAN IMPROVE ON

OTHER COMMENTS

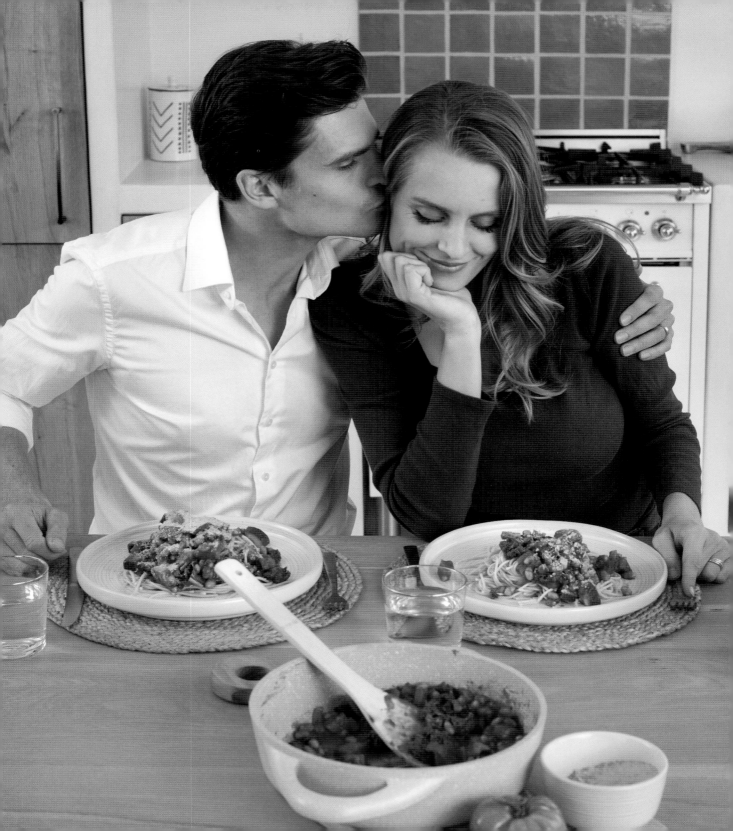

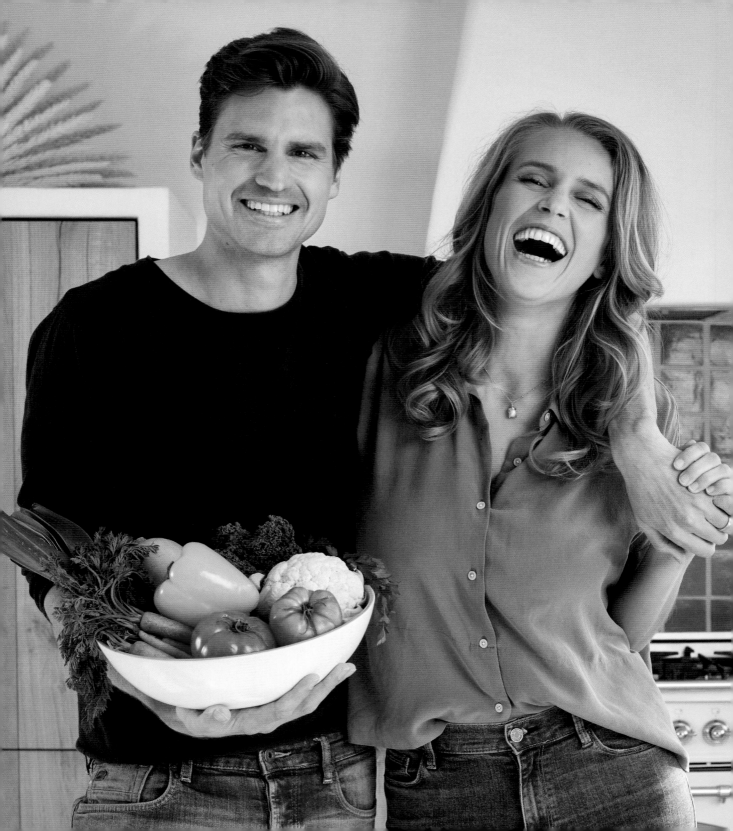

A LAST WORD ON HEALTH

What is your definition of health? Many people define health by the way they look, not eating too much, or losing weight. We want to challenge you to change your definition of health. We want to encourage you to adopt a new way of thinking that health is about feeling good. It's about feeling energetic, balanced, capable, well-rested, pain-free. This approach to health just might also change the world, and that feels good too!

Rethinking the food you eat every day is one highly effective way to be healthier, but being healthy is about more than just food. Here are some of our general, easy tips that will help you optimize your health, so you can feel like the best, most energetic version of yourself.

We focus on eight key areas of health:

- **PLANT-BASED FOOD:** Eating lots and lots of plants is the foundation for feeling healthy and having the energy to live your fullest life.
- **MOVING YOUR BODY DAILY**: Whether it's going for a walk, doing some yoga and Pilates or breaking a sweat with high-intensity training, sports, or running, make sure you move daily.
- **DRINKING CLEAN WATER:** Our bodies are 60 percent water! We recommend using a water filter. Water filtration removes impurities and dangerous contaminants such as chlorine, disinfection by-products, and heavy metals like mercury, lead, and arsenic. There are many good options out there—we use a Berkey water filter on the counter or you can choose to install a filter below the counter. And drink enough of it! About eight 8-ounce glasses, which is about half a gallon a day. Many people are dehydrated and don't realize it.
- **FRESH AIR:** Air quality matters. Go outside and enjoy nature often. We all need more of it. Take a deep breath in the fresh air.
- **A MINDFULNESS PRACTICE:** There are many benefits of meditation, including reducing stress, lowering anxiety, improving sleep, reducing blood pressure, and increasing attention span.[1] Find your way to connect with yourself and make it a routine.
- **HEALTHY RELATIONSHIPS:** Your relationships with the people around you matter. Spend time with the people you love and communicate openly.
- **YOUR PURPOSE AND MISSION IN LIFE:** Find and do something you love and truly care about. Find joy in your work and everything else you do.
- **SLEEP AND REST:** Sleep seven to eight hours whenever you can. Sleep in a dark room. We all make better decisions when we feel rested.

Support and Connect

 We are here for you! Three years ago we started **Your Super Podcast** where we discuss all aspects of health and wellness from a holistic perspective, such as plant-based eating, mindfulness, and natural healing. Everyone has their own journey going plant-based, and as you are about to embark on yours, it can help you to hear about others'.

If you have questions or want to learn more about Your Super way of eating, connect with us and the community on **kristelandmichael.com** as well on our Instagram **@kristelandmichael**. We love connecting with people and also would love to hear your success story!

OLD BELIEFS	TRUE HEALTH
Standard Western diet	Plant-based diet
Absence of disease	Full of energy
Calorie restriction	Eating an abundance of whole plant-based foods
Strict rules	Intuitive eating
Low carbs/no sugar	Eat carbs and sugar from whole foods
Weight loss	True health
All or nothing (start on Monday again)	It's not about being perfect
Diets	Changing habits long-term
Pressure of looking thin	Feeling good and healthy!
Pop a pill	Food as medicine
Depriving	Fueling
Move your body to lose weight as a punishment	Want to move to get blood flowing and feel good
Skinny and tired	High-energy, healthy-looking strong body
Moody and depressed	Sense of joy and fulfillment; able to concentrate
Read nutrition label	Read ingredient list

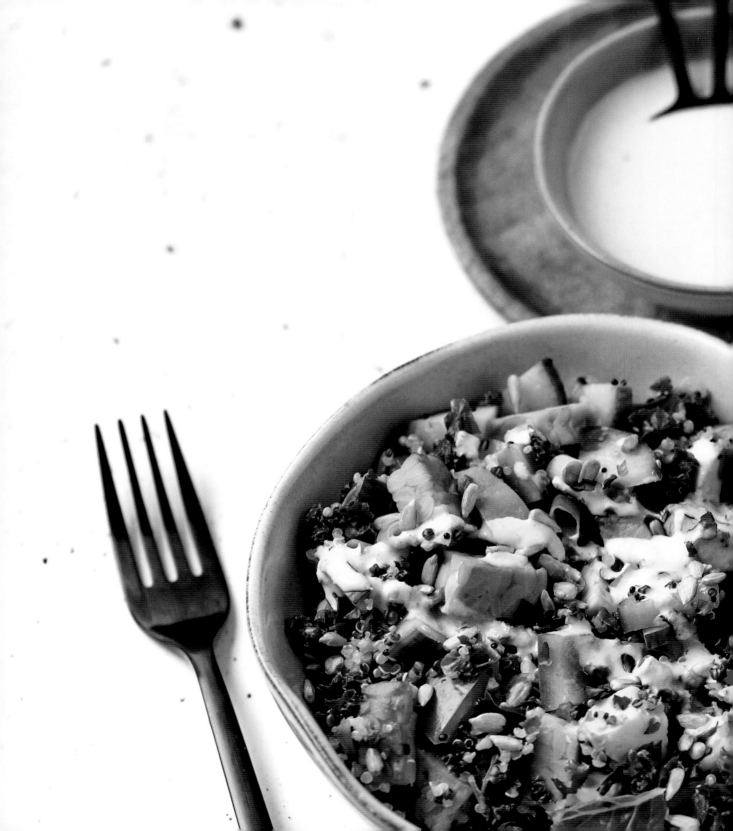

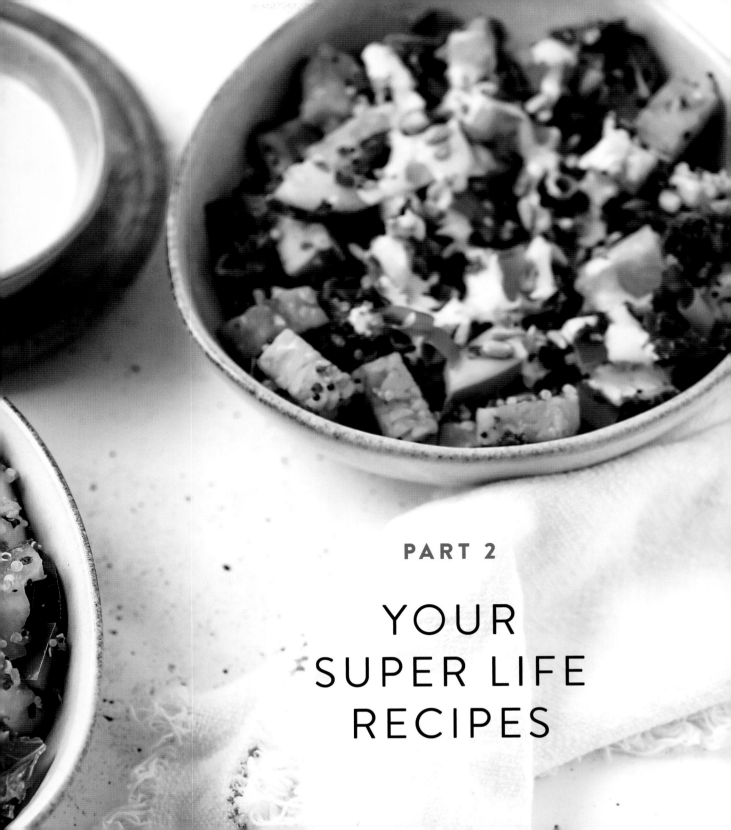

PART 2

YOUR
SUPER LIFE
RECIPES

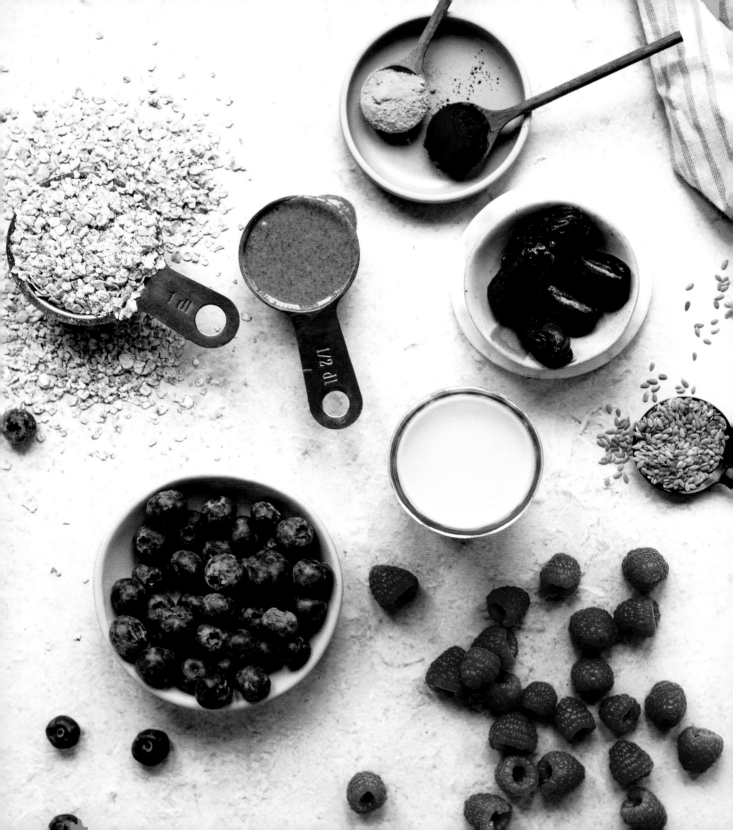

UPLIFT
BUILD A BETTER BREAKFAST

Mornings set the tone for your day. Some say that your body absorbs the most nutrients during breakfast as it comes after the overnight fast. It's the perfect way to start supporting your body and mood for the day by eating fruits, veggies, and superfoods.

Many of the recipes can be prepped the night before so they don't require a lot of extra time in the morning. Starting your morning with superfood-filled smoothies, bowls, and oatmeal keeps you full longer and gives you energy all morning long, .

We'll also teach you the best superfoods to add for what you need: like antioxidant skin boosters açaí and maqui and green superfoods like wheatgrass, spirulina, and moringa. And we break down how to build your perfect overnight oats, smoothies, and açaí bowls.

We encourage you to drink water first thing in the morning to hydrate. Then we like to move our bodies in the morning, whether it's 15 minutes of Pilates, a walk while listening to a podcast, or going for a run. From there it's time for breakfast, something we do our best to make time for, even if we have a million places to rush off to.

As with all meals, choosing breakfast is all about listening to your body. What do you feel like having? This may change seasonally: In the summer months you may want a refreshing smoothie, while in the winter you may crave something warmer. Listen to your body and give it what it needs.

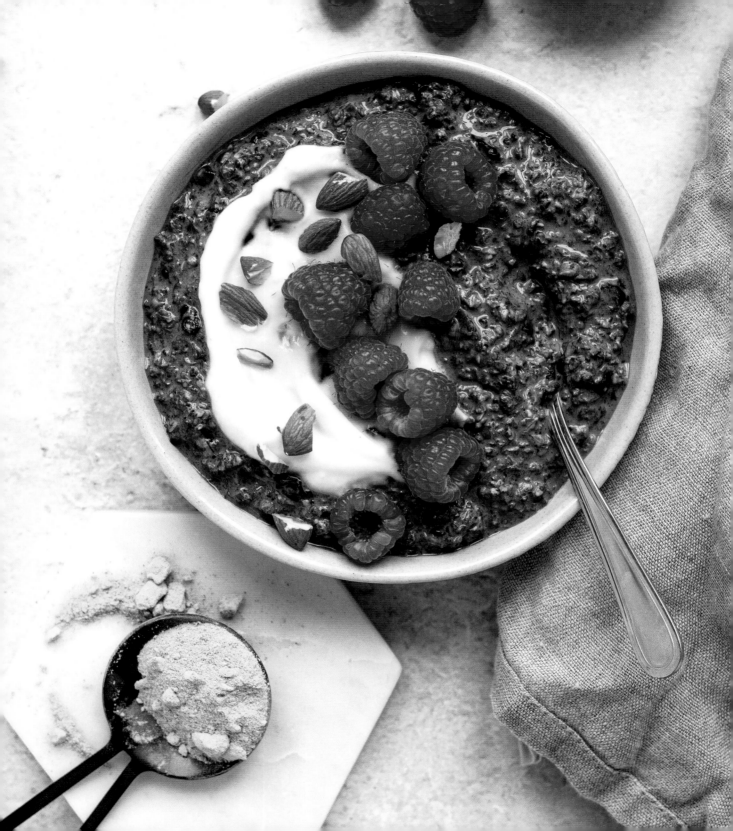

BERRY OATS OVERNIGHT
HEALTHY SKIN & HORMONE HEALTH

SERVES 1 • Overnight oats are perfect when you don't have a lot of time for breakfast, because you do all the work the night before. You can even pop them in a to-go container on busy mornings. These overnight oats are filling and full of fiber. They can also include açaí powder and tocos to support skin health; chia seeds for powerful antioxidants; and omega-3 and vitamin E for skin health as well as the hormone-balancing adaptogen maca.

1 cup quick oats

1 cup oat milk

⅓ cup frozen blueberries

2 tablespoons raisins

2 teaspoons tocos powder, optional

1 teaspoon açaí powder

1 teaspoon chia seeds, optional

½ teaspoon maca powder, optional

TOPPINGS (OPTIONAL)

1 tablespoon almond butter

1 tablespoon cashews

1 tablespoon shredded coconut

1 teaspoon cacao nibs

½ banana, sliced

½ cup mixed berries

COMBINE all ingredients in a bowl or container. Stir to combine. Cover and place in the fridge for 15 minutes or overnight.

IN the morning, add your favorite toppings and enjoy!

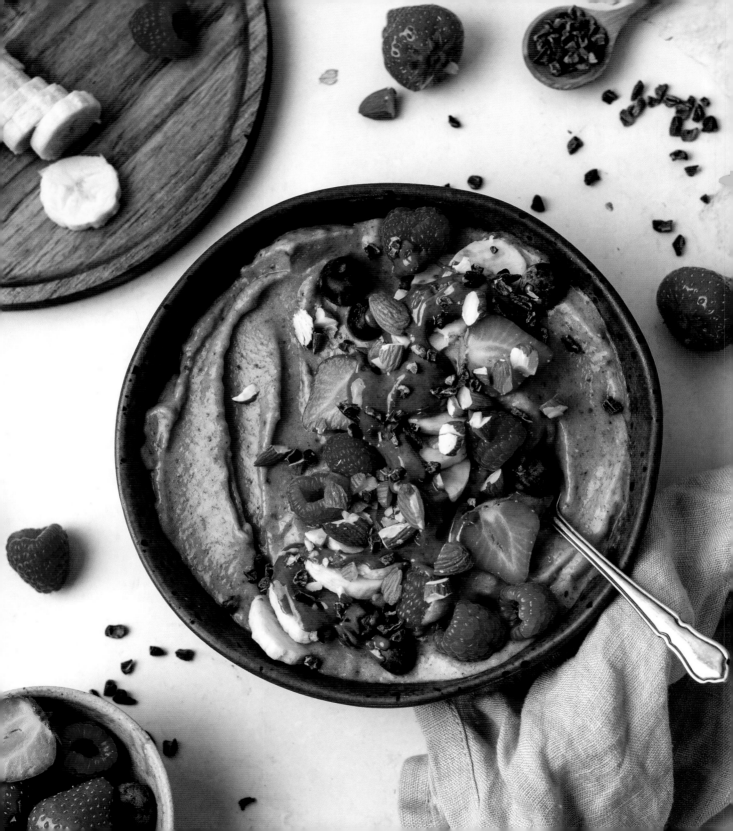

EASY AÇAÍ BOWL
HEALTHY SKIN & ENERGY

SERVES 1 • Any smoothie can become a smoothie bowl by using less liquid and garnishing with your favorite toppings for a little crunch. This is one of our favorites because it includes the mighty combination of açaí and maqui so it's loaded with skin-loving antioxidants. Açaí berries are a Brazilian superfruit native to the Amazon region. Açaí berries are half-inch-round fruits that grow on açaí palm trees. They have dark purple skin and yellow flesh surrounding a large seed. Açaí berries boast three times the amount of antioxidants found in blueberries! Add guarana for an extra energy boost as it contains long-lasting, slowly released caffeine. If your blender struggles to get everything smooth, you can add more liquid—it will just make it a little thinner and less creamy.

1 frozen banana

1 cup frozen strawberries

½ cup frozen cauliflower florets

2 teaspoons açaí powder

1 teaspoon maqui powder, optional

½ teaspoon guarana powder, optional

½ cup canned coconut milk

TOPPINGS (OPTIONAL)

1 tablespoon nut butter

½ banana, sliced

½ cup mixed berries

1 tablespoon shredded coconut

1 teaspoon cacao nibs

1 tablespoon chopped almonds

PLACE all smoothie ingredients in a high-speed blender and puree until smooth. Add more coconut milk, if needed, to blend.

POUR the smoothie into a bowl and garnish with toppings of your choice.

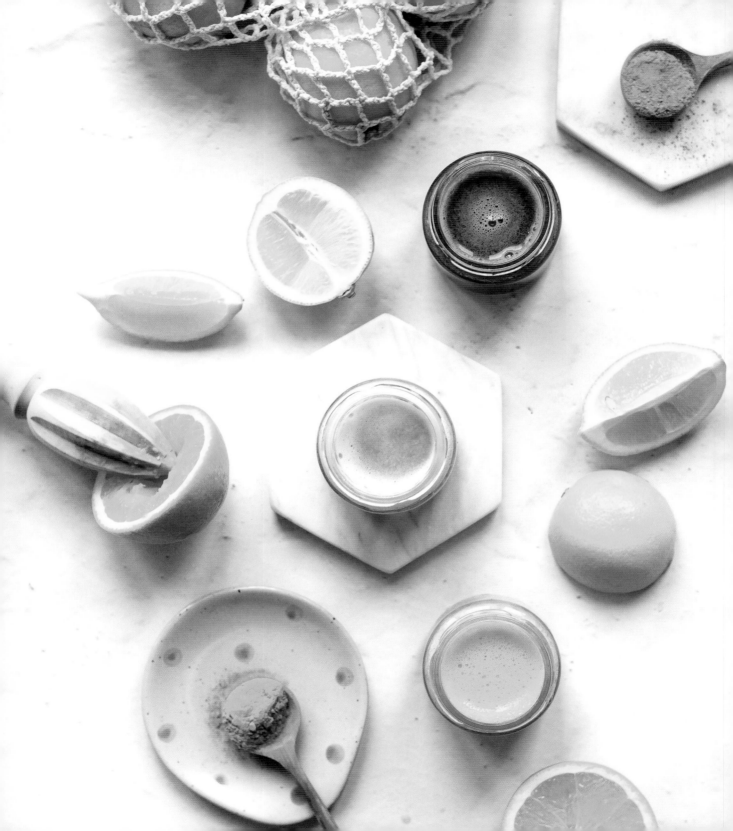

MORNING SHOTS

DETOX & IMMUNITY & ANTI-INFLAMMATORY & HORMONE HEALTH

SERVES 1 • These quick morning shots are our favorite way to get our daily dose of superfoods. Use coconut water instead of plain cold water for an extra burst of flavor. They are easy to take along with any breakfast and are perfect when you are on the go or traveling and can't blend up a whole smoothie.

DETOX SHOT | DETOX & IMMUNITY

1 teaspoon wheatgrass powder

1 teaspoon spirulina powder, optional

1 teaspoon chlorella powder, optional

Juice of ½ lemon

1 cup filtered water or coconut water

TURMERIC SHOT | ANTI-INFLAMMATORY & IMMUNITY

½ teaspoon turmeric powder

½ teaspoon ginger powder

1 teaspoon acerola powder, optional

Juice of ½ fresh orange

1 cup filtered water or coconut water

HORMONE BOOSTER SHOT | HORMONE HEALTH

½ teaspoon maca powder

½ teaspoon shatavari powder, optional

2 teaspoons baobab powder

1 cup filtered water or coconut water

COMBINE all ingredients and stir well with a fork (or put it all in a small container with a lid and shake). Take the shot right away.

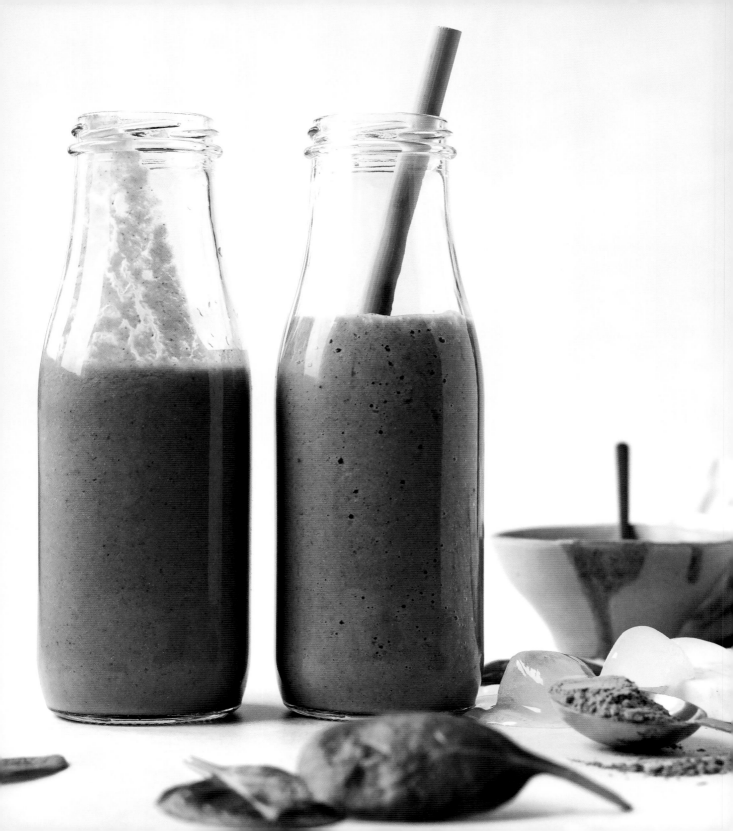

CLASSIC GREEN SMOOTHIE
DETOX & IMMUNITY

SERVES 1 • Green superfoods are powerful for detoxing, immunity, and your overall health. Moringa is a plant that has been praised for its health benefits for thousands of years. The leaves of this native plant of India contain all essential vitamins and minerals, including protein, vitamin A, vitamin B_6, vitamin C, riboflavin, and iron. We keep frozen banana slices in the freezer for making smoothies super fast. To freeze, cut a ripe banana (the riper the sweeter) into five slices and place on a plate in the freezer overnight (so they don't freeze stuck together), then transfer to a sealed container and store in the freezer. Frozen bananas make smoothies rich and creamy. If it's cold outside and you don't want to drink something really cold, use fresh banana and spinach instead of frozen.

1 frozen banana

½ cup frozen spinach

1 tablespoon almond butter

1 teaspoon wheatgrass powder

1 teaspoon chlorella powder, optional

1 teaspoon spirulina powder, optional

1 teaspoon moringa powder, optional

THROW all ingredients in a high-speed blender with 1½ cups of water. Blend until smooth.

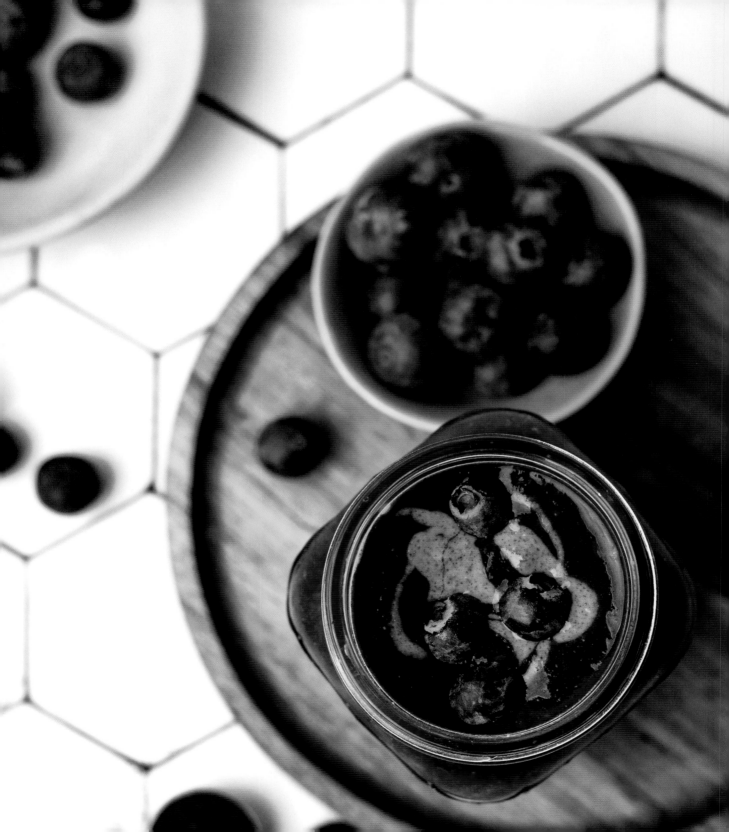

PROTEIN BERRY SMOOTHIE

HEALTHY SKIN & PLANT PROTEIN

SERVES 1 • Hemp is a high-quality vegan protein, containing all nine essential amino acids, plus fiber, healthy fats, and minerals. Like any plant-based protein it's very easy to digest and absorb. Hemp protein powder contains omega-6 and omega-3 fats in an ideal 3:1 ratio. It is also a very sustainable protein—with its deep, strong roots, hemp replenishes the soil with far more nutrients than it uses up. In this smoothie, we combine hemp with delicious antioxidant-rich berries and creamy almond butter for a filling, skin-nourishing meal or snack.

1 cup frozen blueberries

1 pitted date

1 tablespoon almond butter

2 tablespoons hemp protein powder, optional

1 teaspoon açaí powder

1 teaspoon maqui powder, optional

COMBINE all ingredients in a high-speed blender with 1½ cups of water and blend until smooth.

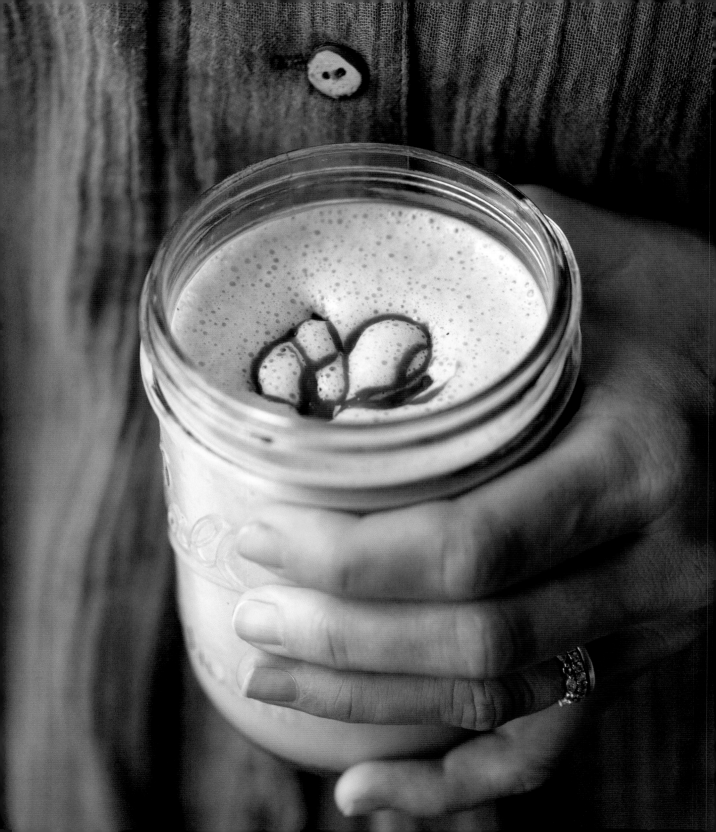

PEANUT PROTEIN SMOOTHIE

HORMONE HEALTH & PLANT PROTEIN

SERVES 1 • Shatavari and maca are both adaptogens that support hormone health. Shatavari has been used for centuries in India for female health and fertility. It can be extremely beneficial for women's reproductive health throughout all life stages. Benefits include increased breast milk production, nourishing the reproductive organs, strengthening female fertility, and providing nourishment to the mother and fetus during pregnancy. It has even been linked to stabilizing one's mood and emotions during the menstrual cycle. Together with banana, peanut butter, and pea protein powder, shatavari and maca make this smoothie filling and hormone balancing.

1 frozen banana

½ cup frozen cauliflower florets, optional

1 tablespoon peanut butter

2 tablespoons pea protein powder

½ teaspoon shatavari powder, optional

1 teaspoon maca powder

1 cup oat milk

PLACE all ingredients in a high-speed blender and process until smooth.

CHOCOLATE PROTEIN SMOOTHIE

MOOD BOOSTER & HEALTHY FATS

SERVES 1 • Why not start your day with chocolate? Cacao powder is made of fermented cacao beans, so you're basically eating a vegetable. You can also add chaga to this smoothie for extra antioxidants. In addition to regulating the immune system, the types of beta-D-glucans found in chaga have been shown to help lower blood sugar levels. We also love adding some frozen cauliflower to our smoothies. Cauliflower is a cruciferous vegetable that is naturally high in fiber and B vitamins. It provides antioxidants and phytonutrients that can protect against cancer. It also contains fiber for healthy digestion.

½ avocado

3 pitted dates

½ cup frozen cauliflower

2 teaspoons cacao powder

½ teaspoon chaga powder, optional

2 tablespoons pea protein powder

1 teaspoon flaxseeds, optional

1½ cups almond milk

PLACE all ingredients in a high-speed blender and process until smooth.

OATGURT WITH APPLE

PLANT PROTEIN

SERVES 1 • We realize that "oatgurt" is not technically a term, but it accurately describes this yummy oat milk yogurt Kristel makes when we are out of almond or coconut yogurt at home. It's an easy way to make a creamy, thick, protein-rich base to enjoy with your favorite fruits, nuts, and seeds. You can even sprinkle superfoods right on top. This is our basic apple cinnamon recipe, but you could do a variation with fresh blueberries and 1 teaspoon açaí powder—or fresh oranges with ½ teaspoon turmeric powder. The possibilities are endless!

1 cup quick oats

1 teaspoon cinnamon powder

1 pitted date

2 tablespoons pea protein powder

2 teaspoons tocos powder, optional

TOPPINGS

1 diced apple

1 tablespoon almond butter, optional

1 tablespoon walnuts

COMBINE the oats, cinnamon, date, protein powder, and tocos, if using, in a large bowl. Add 1 cup of water and stir well to make sure the oats are wet. Cover and let soak for two hours or in the refrigerator overnight.

AFTER soaking, pour mixture into a blender and process until you've got a smooth, thick mixture.

POUR into a bowl and top with apple, almond butter, if using, and walnuts.

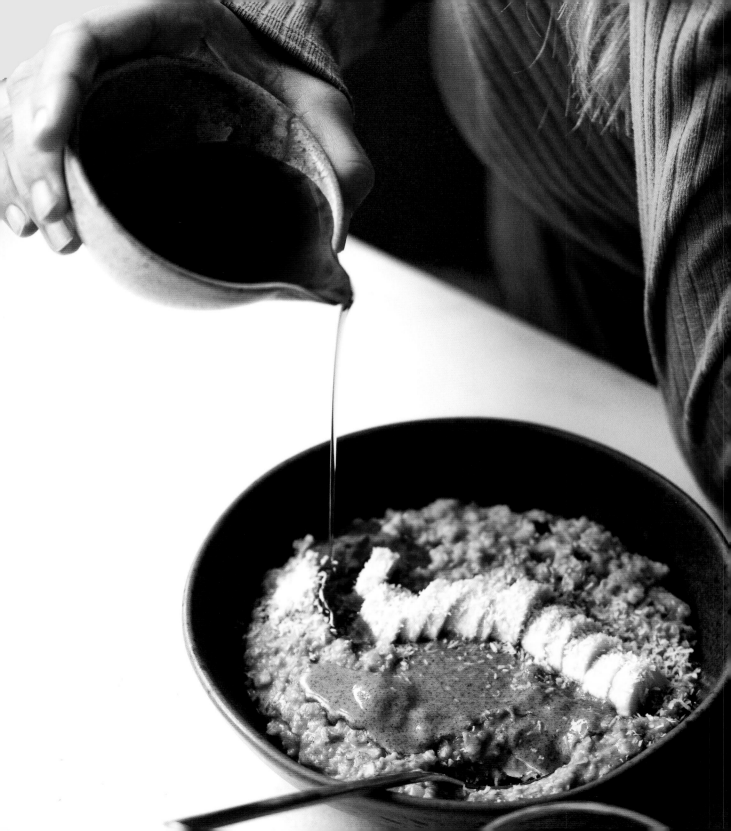

CREAMY TURMERIC OATS
ANTI-INFLAMMATORY & IMMUNITY

SERVES 1 • Oats are among the healthiest grains on earth. They're rich in carbs and fiber, but also higher in protein and fat than most other grains. They are very high in many vitamins and minerals—including manganese, phosphorus, magnesium, copper, iron, zinc, folate, and other B vitamins. They also contain many powerful antioxidants, including avenanthramides. Coconut cream is the thick part on top of the coconut milk can. It makes your oats extra creamy and adds healthy fats. Did you know fats can support the absorption of nutrients of the foods you are eating?

1 cup quick oats

½ banana, sliced

½ teaspoon turmeric powder

½ teaspoon tulsi powder, optional

½ teaspoon ginger powder

1 teaspoon cinnamon powder

2 tablespoons raisins

½ cup canned coconut milk

TOPPINGS (OPTIONAL)

1 tablespoon almond butter

1 tablespoon shredded coconut

½ sliced banana

COMBINE oats, banana, turmeric, tulsi, if using, ginger, cinnamon, raisins, and coconut cream with 1½ cups of water in a small pot.

COOK over medium heat for 5 to 10 minutes, stirring often to prevent burning or sticking, until thick and creamy. Add more water if it gets too thick. Remove from heat.

POUR into a bowl and top with almond butter, shredded coconut, and sliced banana. Serve immediately.

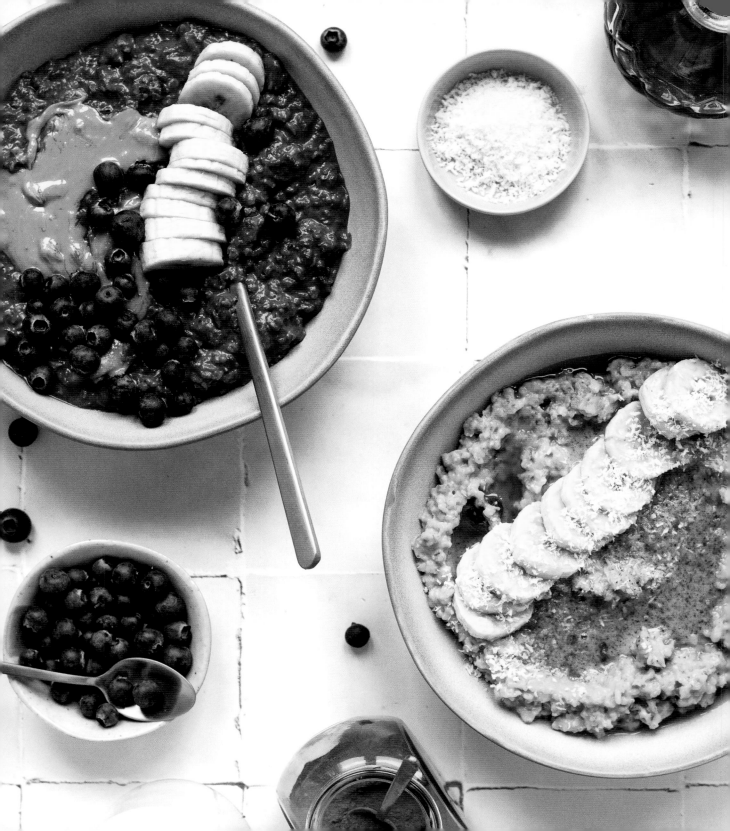

MAGIC CHOCO OATS
MOOD BOOSTER & HEALTHY FATS

SERVES 1 • These indulgent chocolate oats keep you full for a long time, with added superfoods like flaxseeds. Flaxseeds are rich in the omega-3 fatty acid ALA, lignans, and fiber, and can be used to improve digestive health. ALA is one of the two essential fatty acids that you have to obtain from the food you eat, as your body doesn't produce them. Here we add them to oats but they work just as well in smoothies.

1 cup quick oats

1½ cups almond milk

2 teaspoons cacao powder

½ teaspoon reishi powder, optional

1 teaspoon flaxseeds, optional

3 pitted dates, sliced

½ banana, sliced

TOPPINGS (OPTIONAL)

½ banana

1 tablespoon peanut butter

⅓ cup blueberries

COMBINE oats, almond milk, cacao, reishi and flaxseeds, if using, dates, and banana in a small pot.

COOK over medium heat, stirring often to prevent burning or sticking, for 5 to 10 minutes. Add more water if the mixture gets too thick.

REMOVE from heat and pour into a bowl. Add toppings, if desired, and serve.

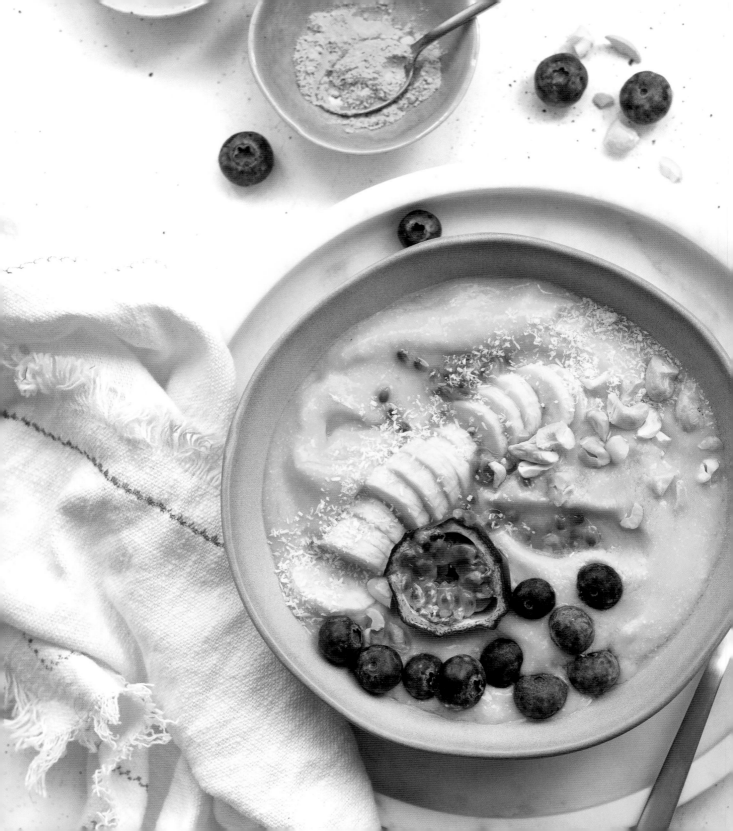

TROPICAL YELLOW SMOOTHIE BOWL

ANTI-INFLAMMATORY & IMMUNITY

SERVES 1 • This refreshing smoothie bowl is absolutely loaded with vitamin C. Mango and pineapple both boost your immunity—they are also both high in fiber and digestive enzymes that will support your digestion. About one gram of acerola cherry powder includes a full serving of daily vitamin C too. Besides boosting your immunity, vitamin C supports your body to produce more collagen, which aids immunity, iron absorption, and cell growth and repair. Turmeric and ginger root are both traditionally used in the ancient Indian healing tradition of Ayurveda for anti-inflammation.

½ cup canned coconut milk

1 cup frozen mango

½ cup frozen pineapple

½ teaspoon turmeric powder

½ teaspoon ginger powder

1 teaspoon acerola powder, optional

TOPPINGS (OPTIONAL)

1 tablespoon chopped raw cashews

1 tablespoon shredded coconut

1 passion fruit, halved and spooned out

PLACE coconut milk, mango, pineapple, turmeric, ginger, and acerola in a high-speed blender and process until smooth.

POUR into a bowl and top with cashews, shredded coconut, and passion fruit, or your favorite toppings.

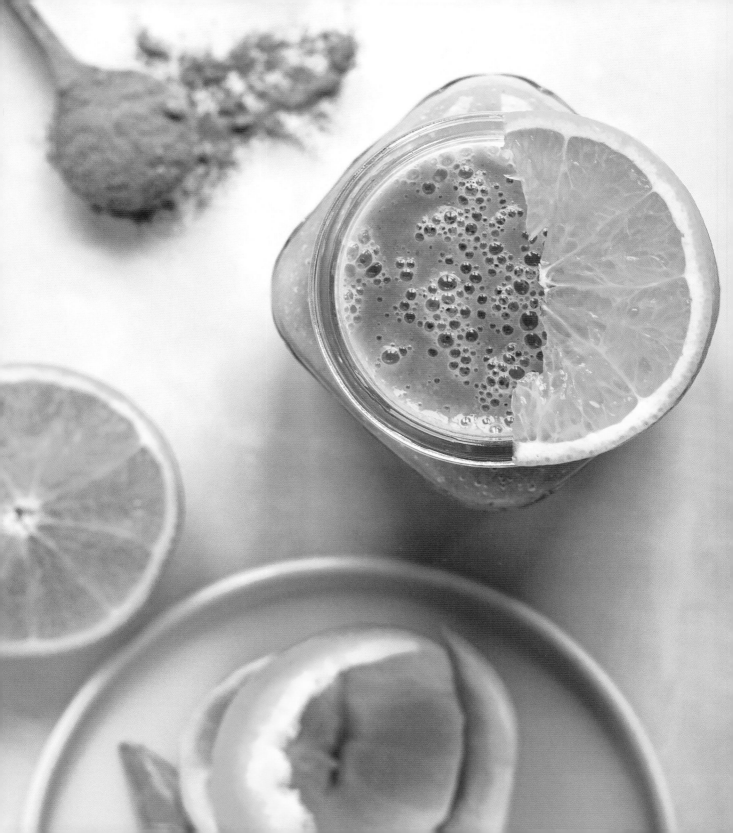

FRUITY GREEN SMOOTHIE
DETOX & IMMUNITY

SERVES 1 • Green smoothies are a brilliant way to load up on all the greens first thing in the morning—feels like winning! You can add all the green superfoods you like to this recipe, whatever you can find in your kitchen cabinet—you can even make a mixture of all your favorite green superfood powders so you can easily add them to your favorite bowls and smoothies. Spirulina is an organism that grows in both fresh and salt water. Gram for gram, spirulina may be the single most nutritious food on the planet. It has 4 grams of protein per 7 grams or about 2 teaspoons. It's a good source of B vitamins, copper, iron, and decent amounts of magnesium, potassium, manganese, and small amounts of almost every other nutrient that you need. It is a type of cyanobacteria, a family of single-celled microbes that are often referred to as blue-green algae. Spirulina was consumed by the ancient Aztecs but became popular again when NASA proposed that it could be grown in space for use by astronauts. Pay attention to what your spirulina smells like—a good source won't smell or taste fishy.

½ head romaine lettuce, chopped

⅓ cucumber

1 frozen banana

1 orange, peeled

1 teaspoon wheatgrass powder

1 teaspoon chlorella powder, optional

1 teaspoon spirulina powder, optional

1 teaspoon moringa powder, optional

1 cup ice cubes, optional

COMBINE all ingredients with 1½ cups water in a high-speed blender and process until smooth.

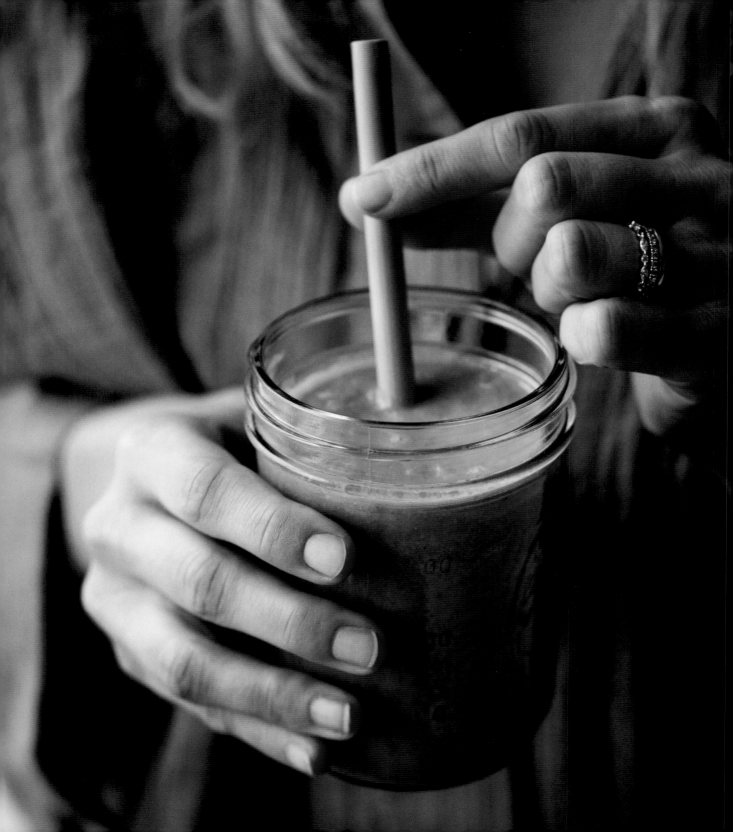

ALL-GREEN SMOOTHIE
DETOX & IMMUNITY

SERVES 1 • Here's an all-green smoothie if you like it green and a little mean. Play around with this and feel free to add all the green superfoods. If it ends up too green and bitter, you can always sweeten it up with 1 or 2 pitted dates, a little lime or lemon juice, or fresh mint leaves. In any green smoothie, try switching it up and using a variety of leafy greens in your smoothies throughout the week. Kale, spinach, romaine, herbs, and carrot tops are all great options. This way you feed your body a wide variety of nutrients.

½ cucumber

½ cup frozen spinach

½ avocado

½ lime, peeled

½ teaspoon ginger powder

2 tablespoons hemp protein powder, optional

1 teaspoon wheatgrass powder

1 teaspoon baobab powder, optional

1 cup ice cubes, optional

COMBINE all the ingredients with 1 cup of water in a high-speed blender and process until smooth.

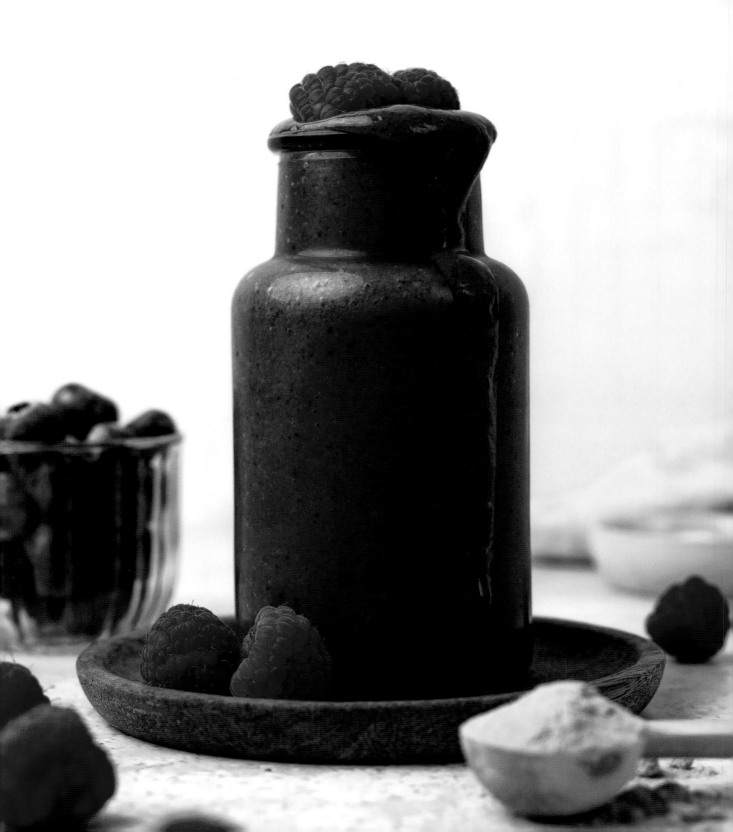

BERRY HORMONE SMOOTHIE

HEALTHY SKIN & HORMONE HEALTH

SERVES 1 • Maca grows on the mountaintops in Peru where nothing else grows anymore, mainly in the Andes of central Peru, in harsh conditions and at very high altitudes—above 13,000 feet. It is a cruciferous vegetable that's related to broccoli, cauliflower, cabbage, and kale. Maca root has traditionally been used to enhance fertility and sex drive; some people say it gives them a boost of energy. It is sometimes referred to as Peruvian ginseng. It combines with antioxidant-rich berries and healthy fats to make one happy hormone smoothie that your taste buds will love.

½ cup frozen blueberries

½ cup frozen raspberries

1 banana

1 teaspoon açaí powder

1 teaspoon maqui powder, optional

½ teaspoon shatavari powder, optional

½ teaspoon maca powder

⅓ cup canned coconut milk

1½ cups plant-based milk

COMBINE all the ingredients in a high-speed blender and process until smooth.

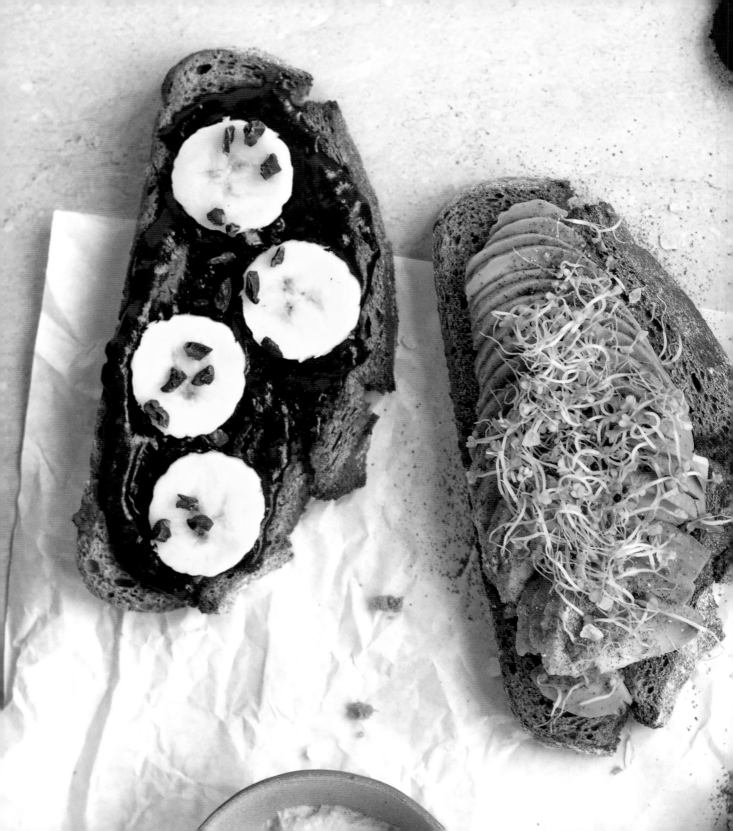

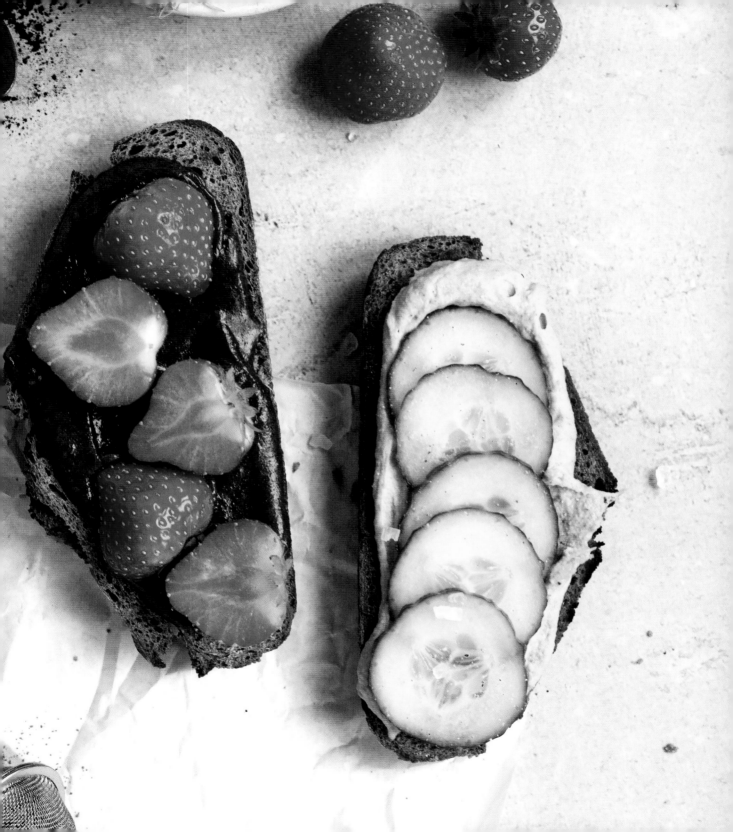

EASY SUPER TOASTS
MOOD BOOSTER & HEALTHY SKIN & DETOX & ENERGY

SERVES 1 • These toasts are a good example of how easy it can be to incorporate superfoods into foods you are probably already eating. We've included four of our favorites, but feel free to be creative with toppings and superfoods to find what you love best. You might use hazelnut butter in place of peanut butter to create an irresistible "Nutella" or swap the açaí powder with turmeric for an anti-inflammatory boost. When choosing a bread make sure to check the ingredient list, as with all packaged products you buy. We love sourdough bread and gluten-free loaves made with oat or buckwheat flour.

INDULGENT PEANUT BUTTER TOAST | MOOD BOOSTER

1 slice bread

3 tablespoons peanut butter

1 teaspoon cacao powder

1 teaspoon maple syrup

1 teaspoon cacao nibs, optional

½ banana, optional

TOAST a slice of bread in a toaster or in the oven until warm and crispy.

MEANWHILE, stir the peanut butter, cacao, and maple syrup together.

WHEN your toast is ready, spread the peanut butter blend over it. Sprinkle the cacao nibs, if using, on top. If you like, garnish with the sliced banana.

ANTIOXIDANT-RICH ALMOND BUTTER TOAST | HEALTHY SKIN

1 slice bread

3 tablespoons almond butter

1 teaspoon açaí powder

3 sliced strawberries, optional

TOAST a slice of bread in a toaster or in the oven until warm and crispy.

MEANWHILE, stir the almond butter and açaí together.

WHEN your toast is ready, spread the almond and açaí butter over it. Garnish with sliced strawberries, if desired.

SUPER GREEN HUMMUS TOAST | DETOX & IMMUNITY

1 slice bread

½ cup hummus

½ teaspoon wheatgrass powder

¼ teaspoon garlic powder

Sea salt and pepper to taste

5 slices cucumber, optional

TOAST a slice of bread in a toaster or in the oven until warm and crispy.

MEANWHILE, combine the hummus, wheatgrass, and garlic powder and stir.

WHEN your toast is ready, spread the hummus over it. Add salt and pepper to taste and garnish with sliced cucumbers, if desired.

ENERGIZING AVO TOAST | ENERGY

1 slice bread

½ avocado

½ teaspoon matcha powder

½ cup alfalfa sprouts, optional

Sea salt and pepper to taste

TOAST a slice of bread in a toaster or in the oven until warm and crispy.

SLICE the avocado and put a single layer on the toasted bread. Sprinkle with matcha powder. Garnish with some alfalfa sprouts, if using. Season with salt and pepper to taste.

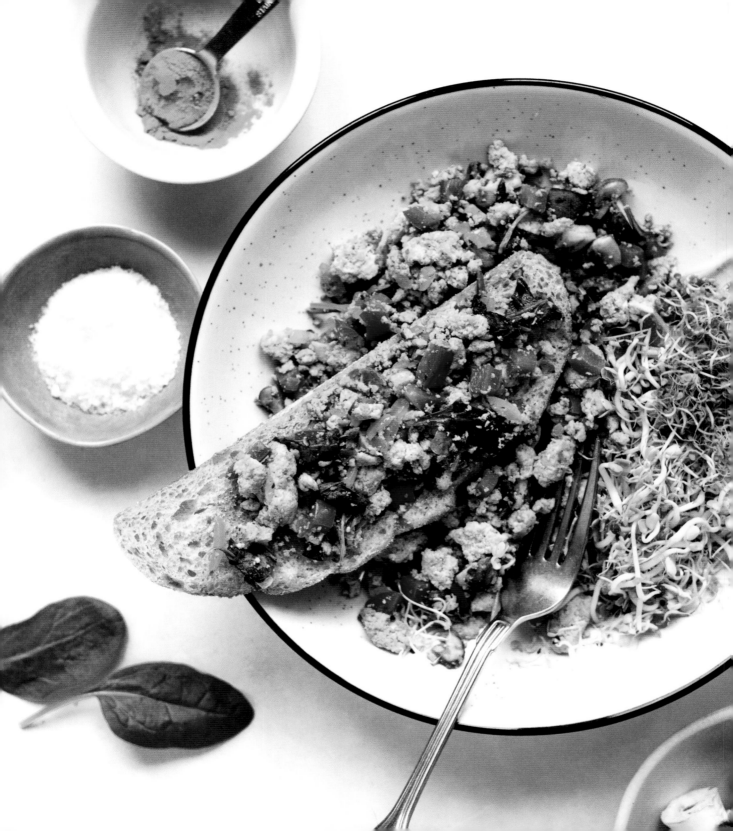

TOFU VEGGIE SCRAMBLE
ANTI-INFLAMMATORY & IMMUNITY

SERVES 1 • Think of this as your healthy version of scrambled eggs. It's especially great for those mornings when you're craving something savory and warm. This dish is great served with reheated leftover potatoes and a slice of toast. Tofu is a complete source of protein, which means it provides all of the essential amino acids needed in the diet. Soybeans are also high in healthy polyunsaturated fats, especially omega-3 alpha-linolenic acid. Made from fermented soy beans, tofu (and soy more broadly) has gotten a bad rap, as some believe it increases estrogen in the body. However, more recent studies show that eating soy foods like tofu, edamame, tempeh, and soy milk have been linked to reduced risk of certain cancers, including breast cancer, prostate cancer, and gastric cancer.[1]

1 cup brown button mushrooms, sliced

½ red bell pepper, sliced

½ small onion, sliced

3 ounces firm tofu, drained and crumbled

1 cup fresh spinach

½ teaspoon turmeric powder

½ teaspoon curry powder

½ teaspoon tulsi powder, optional

½ teaspoon moringa powder, optional

½ teaspoon garlic powder

Sea salt and pepper to taste

1 tablespoon tahini, optional

½ cup alfalfa or broccoli sprouts, optional

HEAT a medium-size ceramic-coated pan over medium-high heat. When the pan is hot, add ¼ cup of water and the mushrooms, red bell pepper, and onions. Sauté until soft, adding more water to prevent sticking to the pan, if needed.

ADD the tofu, spinach, and the turmeric, curry, tulsi, if using, moringa, and garlic powders, and salt and pepper to taste. Stir-fry until veggies soften and the water evaporates.

SERVE immediately, topped with a dollop of tahini and some of your favorite sprouts, if using.

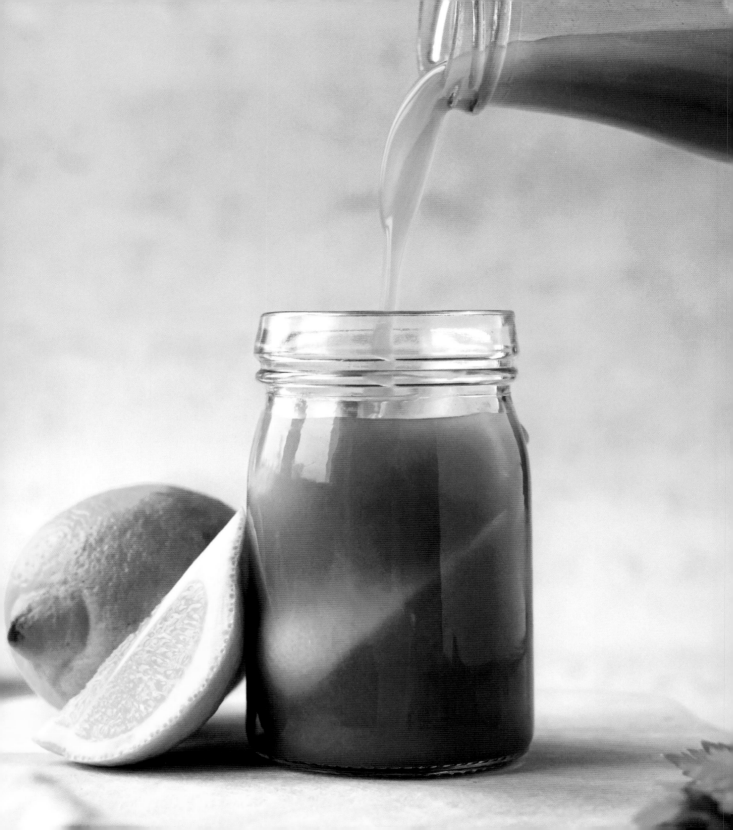

TOTAL GREEN JUICE
DETOX & IMMUNITY

SERVES 1 • This is a hydrating and refreshing juice that's an easy way of getting more greens in the mornings. We recommend a slow juicer rather than a high-speed juicer to get more juice out of your veggies and to maintain more nutrients. Centrifugal juicers work faster because they spin the juice out through a filter with centrifugal force, which needs a lot of speed. Slow juicers use a pressing force to get the juice through the filter without creating too much heat and friction. While it can be tempting to go for the faster juicers, you actually get more juice out of the slow ones!

2 celery stalks

1 cucumber

½ inch fresh ginger root

½ lemon

1 teaspoon wheatgrass powder

1 teaspoon chlorella powder, optional

1 teaspoon spirulina powder, optional

1 teaspoon moringa powder, optional

FOLLOWING your juicer's instructions, juice the celery, cucumber, ginger, and lemon.

STIR in the superfood powders and drink immediately.

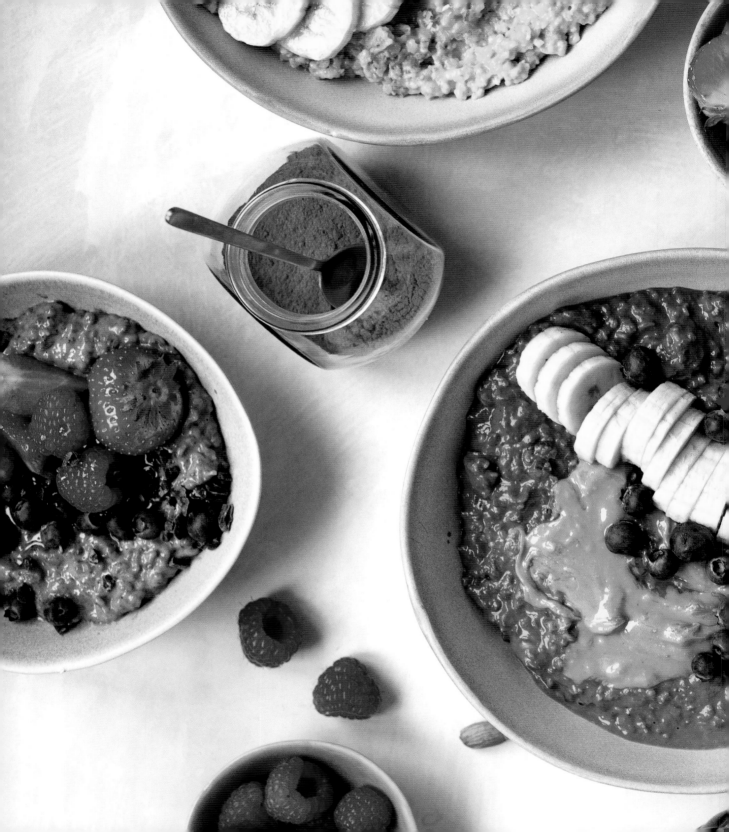

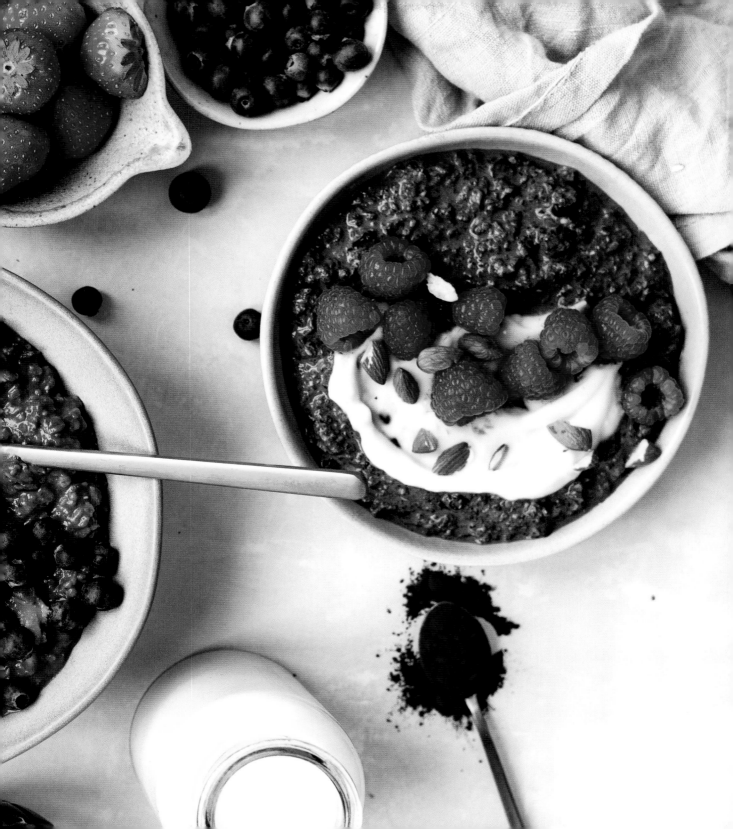

HOW TO MAKE OATMEAL

Oatmeal is so versatile and quick—and rich in fiber, which promotes fullness, eases the insulin response, and benefits gut health. It's also a good source of vitamins B and E and minerals such as magnesium. When you're ready to get creative with your oatmeal, we've got an easy step-by-step plan so that you can create your own unique oatmeal creations. This is a perfect filling breakfast to add your nutritious superfood powders in!

① CHOOSE YOUR OATS

Start with 1 cup of oats. Choose your favorite.

STEEL-CUT OATS: These oats are closest to their original grain form. They are made when the whole groat is cut into several pieces with a steel blade (it looks similar to rice that's been cut into pieces). This variety takes the longest to cook (around 30 minutes) and has a nuttier taste and a chewy texture.

ROLLED OATS: These are whole oats that are first steamed to make them soft and pliable and then rolled to flatten them to a specific thickness. This additional processing means they cook faster (in 2 to 5 minutes). Rolled oats tend to retain their shape when cooked.

QUICK OATS: These are the most processed of the three oat varieties. They are partially cooked, dried, and then rolled and pressed thinner than rolled oats to allow the oats to cook more quickly. Our personal favorite!

② CHOOSE A LIQUID

Choose 1 cup water, almond milk, cashew milk, rice milk, coconut milk, oat milk, or hemp milk.

③ ADD FRUIT

Add fresh, frozen, or dried fruits like banana, apple, berries, raisins, or dates.

④ COOK OR SOAK OVERNIGHT

Heat up your liquid in a saucepan and then add your oats and cook until softened, or to taste. Alternatively, you can combine your oats and liquid in a sealed glass jar overnight; in the morning, they'll be ready to eat as is or warmed up.

⑤ ADD YOUR SUPERFOODS

Add 2 to 3 teaspoons of your favorite superfood powders or superfood mixes. Experiment with different combinations to discover what you like best.

⑥ TOPPINGS!

Add a spoonful of nut butter, shredded coconut, maple syrup, cinnamon, vanilla extract, or chopped nuts.

TIPS

MAKE your oats ahead for a grab-and-go breakfast! Mix all the ingredients together in a mason jar. Cover and refrigerate overnight. Enjoy cold—or heat up in a pot on the stove in the morning!

WHEN we're traveling, we'll add all of the ingredients except the liquid to an empty jar. Once we're up in the air or are on the road, we add water and shake it up for a healthy breakfast or snack.

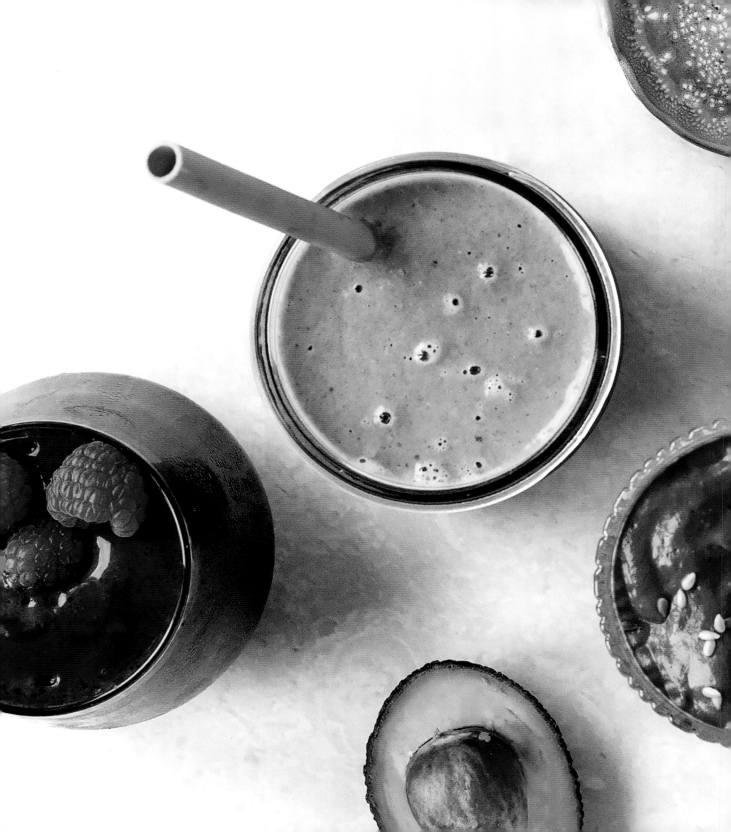

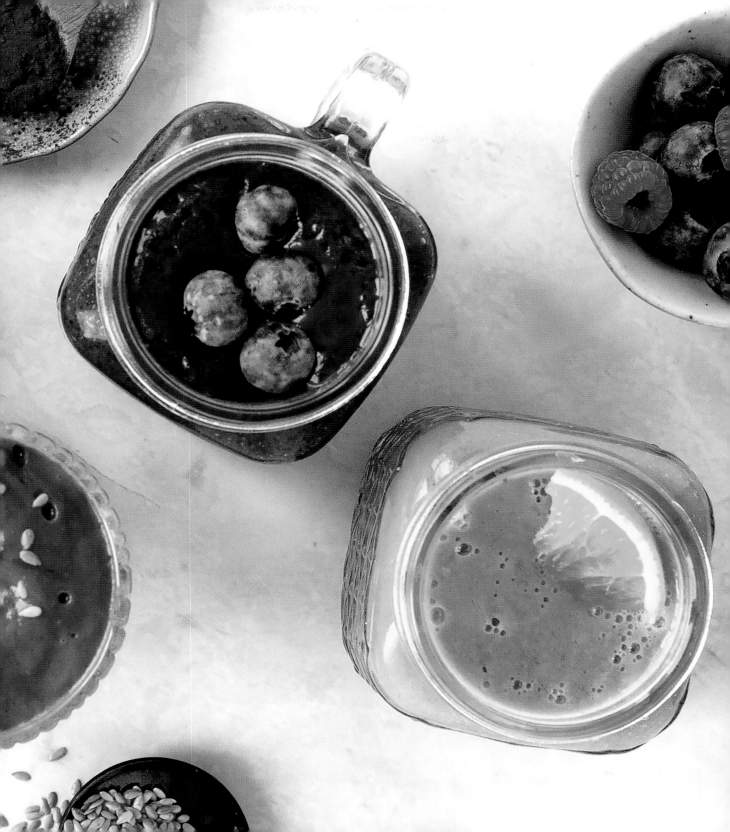

HOW TO BUILD A SMOOTHIE

Smoothies are easy, delicious, and a great way to sneak in extra veggies. We often have them in the morning, but smoothies are also great as an afternoon snack or after a workout. The tricky thing about making your own smoothies is finding the right proportions. This step-by-step guide will help you. Just combine your favorite fruit, veggies, and superfood powders—the options are endless. Have fun finding your favorite combos! Our personal tip is to use a little less liquid so that it's thicker, add toppings, and spoon it out of a bowl. Whether you use fresh or frozen fruit and veggies is up to you—it really just depends whether you prefer a cold smoothie, which is also often more creamy, or a warmer one. The advantage to using frozen is that you always can have them ready to go in the freezer.

① CHOOSE A LIQUID

Start with 1½ cups water or plant-based milk (almond, coconut, and oat work well) or coconut water or fresh juice. You can always add more liquid if you prefer thinner smoothies.

② ADD YOUR SUPERFOODS

Add 3 teaspoons of your favorite superfood powders or mixes. Don't be afraid to experiment to find what works best. Use the superfood table on pages 22 to 23 to find superfoods you currently need most to support your health goals.

③ ADD FRUITS AND VEGGIES

1 TO 2 CUPS FRUIT: Go for your favorites here, and feel free to mix it up and experiment! You can go tropical with mango, pineapple, guava, papaya, passion fruit, and banana. Berries are full of antioxidants: Think strawberries, blueberries, kiwis, raspberries, and blackberries. Citrus fruits like lemon, lime, orange, grapefruit, and clementine make for a fresh and refreshing flavor. Or you can go with classics like apple, pear, dates, nectarine, cherries, and peaches.

1 CUP VEGGIES: Leafy greens such as spinach, romaine lettuce, kale, chard, and celery are great in smoothies. So are veggies like cucumber, zucchini, cauliflower, beets (cooked or raw), carrots, sweet potato (cooked or raw), or avocado.

④ ADD FOR A CREAMY SMOOTHIE

Choose at least one serving of one of the options below to add creaminess to your smoothie. If you already chose banana, avocado, or mango in Step 3 then you don't have to add extra. Options include 1 banana, ½ avocado, 1 cup frozen mango, 1 tablespoon nut butter (such as almond, cashew, peanut, or hazelnut butter), 2 tablespoons plant-based yogurt, 2 tablespoons quick oats, or 2 tablespoons coconut cream.

⑤ BLEND AND ENJOY!

The best smoothies are made in a high-speed blender. Blend for 30 seconds at least. Put in a glass or bowl. Add toppings for an extra crunch if you like. The sky's the limit. Some of our favorites include fruits like apples, bananas, berries, figs, kiwi, mangos, nectarines, pears, passionfruit, or pomegranate. Also think about dried fruits, such as dates, goji, mulberries, or raisins. Nuts and seeds are also a great option: almonds, cashews, hazelnuts, pecans, walnuts, chia, flax, hemp, sesame, or sunflower. Other options include cacao nibs, shredded coconut, nut butter, oats, or granola.

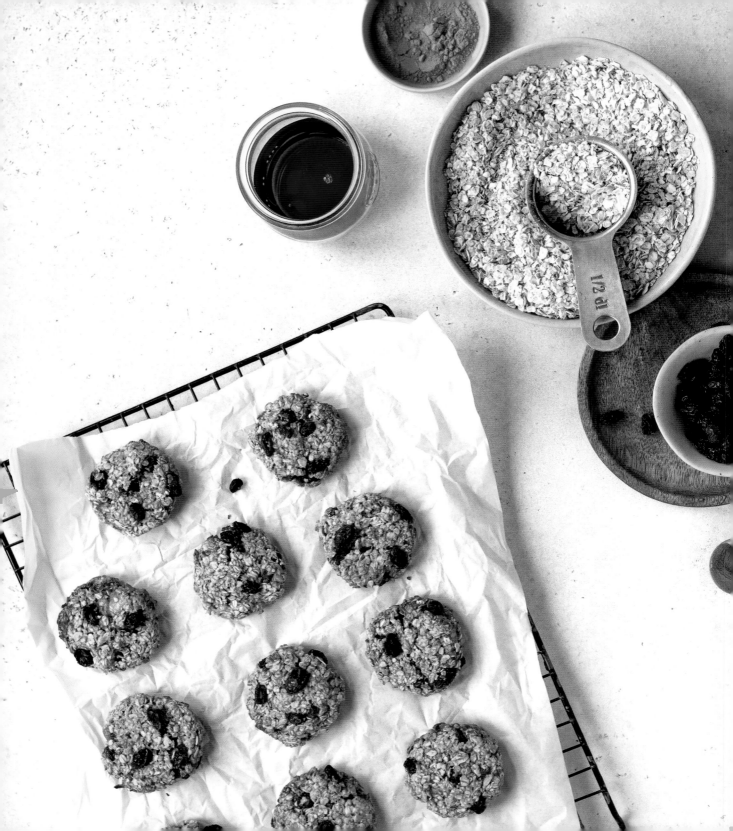

REFRESH

VIBRANT MIDMORNING SNACKS

Unlike many of the popular restrictive fad diets, it's okay to indulge in plant-based snacks! In fact, we highly recommend it. Yes, you read that correctly; you absolutely do not have to deprive yourself of food when you are hungry. The diet industry has taught us to ignore hunger and cravings, emphasizing that "being healthy" is a matter of willpower and deprivation. But if you feel hungry all the time, your body is telling you that you're not giving it the nutrients it needs, and it suggests your blood sugar is unstable. It's also damaging to get into the habit of ignoring your body's signals.

A midmorning snack is a great way to nourish yourself. We love having a morning snack especially if we only had a smoothie earlier, or had to get up super early, or had a big workout in the morning so we feel hungrier. Snacks can also be really beneficial in your diet: They can increase nutrient intake, sustain energy levels, and help your body recover from exercise. You'll find lots of sweet snacks in this chapter as well as recipes with energizing superfoods like guarana, maca, and matcha, and healthy fats and carbs. Think of snacking as an opportunity to get more powerful nutrients in you. We designed these snacks with a focus on high fiber, high protein, and high micronutrients.

If you're a coffee drinker, this is the time of day we'd suggest having it—though we recommend trying one of our energizing superfood lattes instead. They're healthier alternatives to your regular coffee that can give you longer-lasting energy.

Many of these recipes, like our Super Green Balls and Protein Oat Cookies, can be prepped ahead and stored in the fridge so you have them ready when you need them.

We've included a few snack chapters in this book—one for morning snacks, one for afternoon snacks, and one for desserts or light snacks after dinner. You might not need all three every day, and some days you need all of the above. Listen to your body and adjust accordingly.

Not sure if you're really hungry? Have some water. And make sure you're hydrating throughout the day. Sometimes we think we are hungry in between meals when we are truly *thirsty*. You can always make your water special by adding fresh ginger, cucumber, lemon, or lime.

HAPPY HORMONES LATTE
HORMONE HEALTH

1 SERVING • This latte is a little energizing and a little sweet, making it a perfectly comforting midmorning drink—and something to make a daily habit if you struggle with imbalanced hormones, whether they cause PMS, low sex drive, or menopause symptoms. Found in the high mountains of Peru, maca is known for promoting energy, hormone balance, healthy thyroid function, and sexual function and relieving premenstrual syndrome (PMS) and menopause symptoms, among others.[1] If you prefer your lattes iced, simply add ice cubes!

1½ cups plant milk

1 teaspoon maca powder

¼ teaspoon shatavari powder, optional

½ teaspoon cinnamon powder, optional

1 teaspoon maple syrup

WARM up the milk in a small pan on the stove.

ONCE the milk is warm, add maca, shatavari if using, cinnamon if using, and maple syrup. Stir well or use a frother to combine. Enjoy immediately.

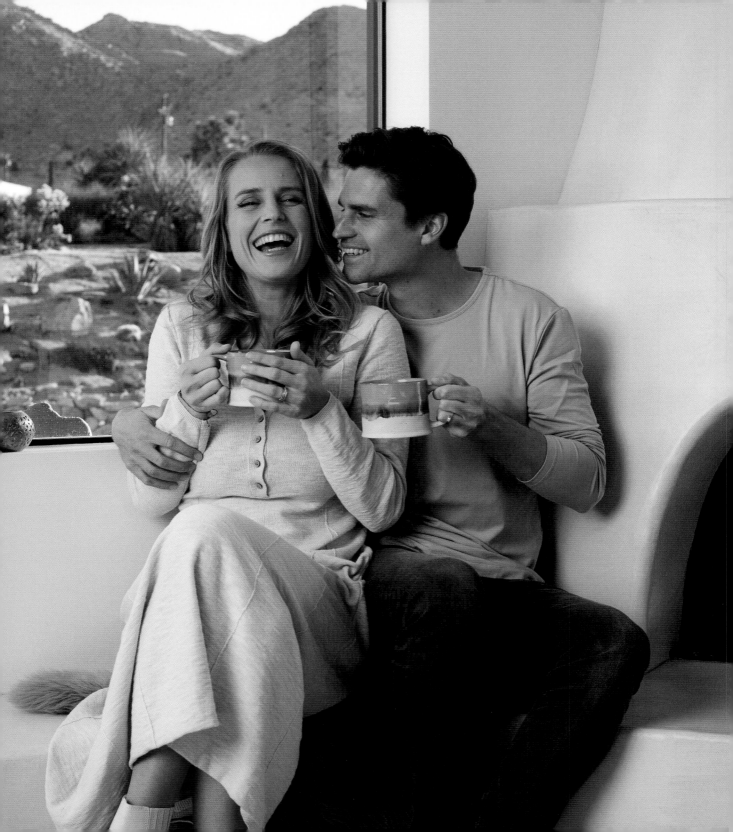

MATCHA LATTE
ENERGY & ANTI-INFLAMMATORY

1 SERVING • Matcha is made of pulverized green tea leaves, originally used by monks in Japan to better concentrate during meditation. The advantage of drinking pulverized tea is that you get all the nutrients in the leaves versus only those that are extracted from steeping your tea bag. Besides caffeine, matcha leaves also contain L-theanine, which helps give you that calm and alert effect.[2] We like to have this midmorning rather than first thing because your body's natural cortisol, which kicks into high gear when you first wake up, makes the first in a series of dips between breakfast and lunch.

1½ cups plant milk

½ teaspoon matcha powder

¼ teaspoon turmeric powder, optional

1 teaspoon maple syrup

WARM the milk in a small saucepan or in a mug.

ONCE the milk is warm, add matcha, turmeric, if using, and maple syrup. Stir or use a frother to combine. Add ice cubes if you prefer an iced latte. Otherwise drink immediately.

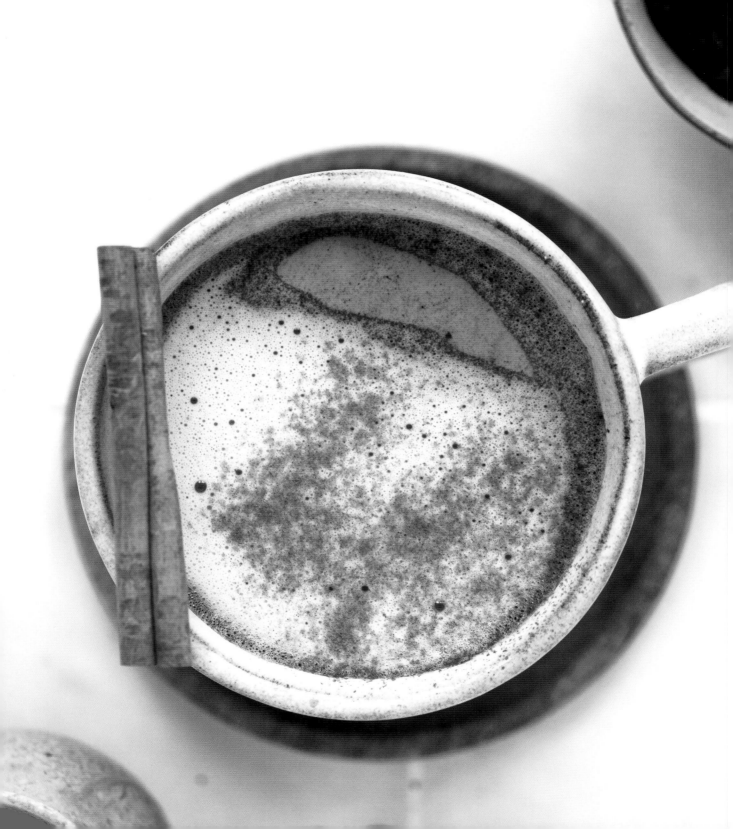

CHAGACHINO

DETOX & IMMUNITY

1 SERVING • Coffee can be acidic and often gives you short-lived, jittery energy. Try replacing it with the immune-system- and energy-boosting chaga mushroom. Be sure to include the guarana for additional long-lasting energy. The guarana vine originated in the Amazon basin, where local people have long taken advantage of its stimulating properties. It's known to reduce fatigue, increase energy, and aid learning and memory. It takes about a week to kick your coffee habit in the butt; chaga and guarana can help!

1½ cups plant milk

1 teaspoon chaga powder

½ teaspoon guarana powder, optional

2 teaspoon tocos powder, optional

1 teaspoon maple syrup

WARM the milk in a small saucepan on the stove or in a mug.

MIX in the chaga, and guarana and tocos, if using, and maple syrup. Stir or use a frother to combine. Enjoy immediately or add ice cubes for an iced latte.

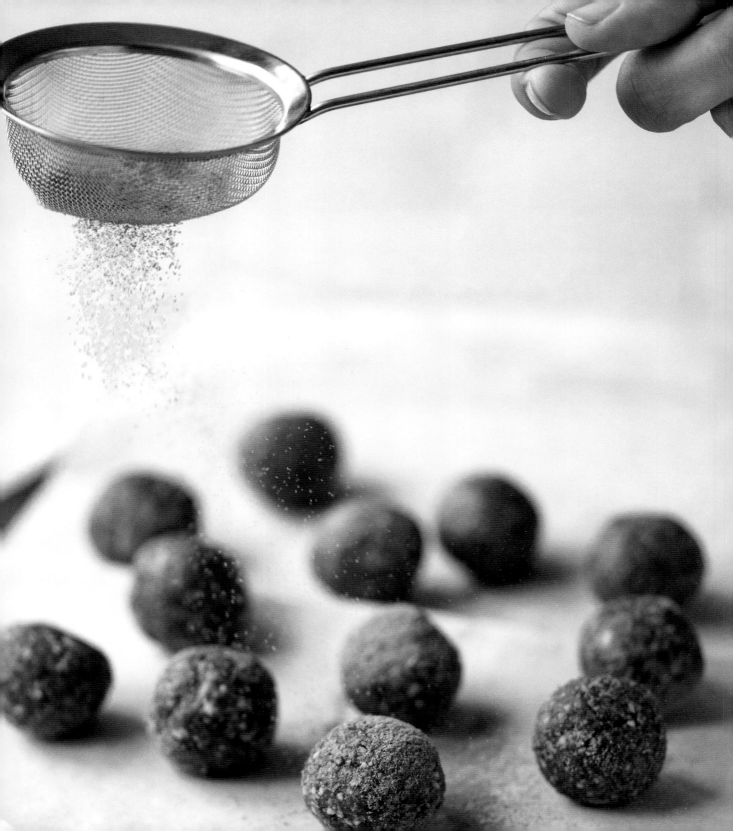

GREEN SUPER BALLS
DETOX & IMMUNITY

4 SERVINGS • This is an easy snack to make ahead and have on hand—we like to keep a batch in the fridge or take it with us on the go. These balls are filling and pack a good punch of greens, something we all always need more of. The wheatgrass alone contains iron, calcium, magnesium, phytonutrients, 17 amino acids, vitamins A, C, E, K, and B complex, and chlorophyll. Nutrient-dense, they support elimination of toxins, digestion, and immunity. Not bad for a quick snack!

1 cup cashews

1 cup dates

Zest and juice of ½ lemon

1 teaspoon wheatgrass powder

1 teaspoon chlorella powder, optional

1 teaspoon moringa powder, optional

BLEND all the ingredients in a high-speed blender until sticky, then roll into 1½-inch balls.

STORE in a sealed container in the refrigerator for 3 to 5 days. Or freeze and store for about three months.

REFRESH

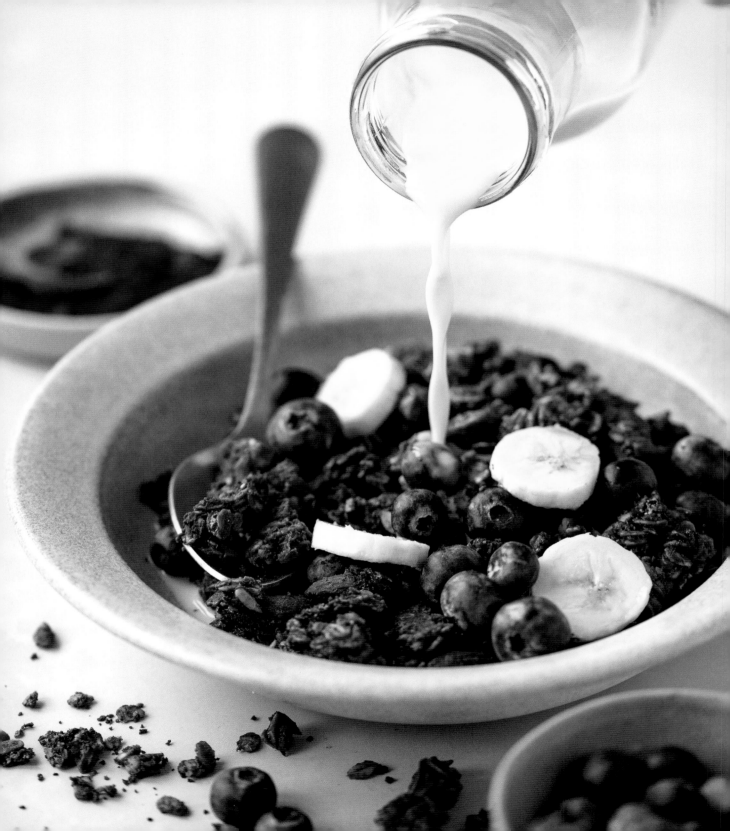

CHOCOLATE GRANOLA

HORMONE HEALTH & MOOD BOOSTER

4 SERVINGS • Store-bought granola tends to have extremely long ingredient lists and lots of sugar. Making it yourself allows you to control what goes in there, which also means you're able to up the nutrition factor with some added superfoods. In this recipe, we include maca and shatavari, the superfoods that support hormone health and mood. This recipe doubles (or even triples) well, so you'll have plenty to eat on its own or sprinkled over plant-based yogurt or milk or even as a garnish, along with sliced bananas and blueberries, on your smoothie bowls.

⅓ cup coconut oil

1½ cups rolled oats

2 tablespoons cacao powder

1 teaspoon maca powder

½ teaspoon shatavari powder, optional

1 teaspoon chia seeds

1 tablespoon sunflower seeds

1 cup almonds

2 tablespoons peanut butter

⅓ cup maple syrup

PREHEAT the oven to 360°F.

IF your coconut oil is solid, melt it in a saucepan and set aside.

MIX all the dry ingredients—oats, cacao, maca, shatavari, if using, chia seeds, sunflower seeds, and almonds—in a large bowl.

ADD the wet ingredients—peanut butter, maple syrup, and the melted coconut oil—and stir well to combine.

SPREAD the mixture out on a parchment-lined baking tray.

BAKE for 25 minutes until crispy, stirring halfway through so it bakes evenly. Let cool and enjoy!

COOL and store in a sealed container at room temperature or in fridge for up to one week.

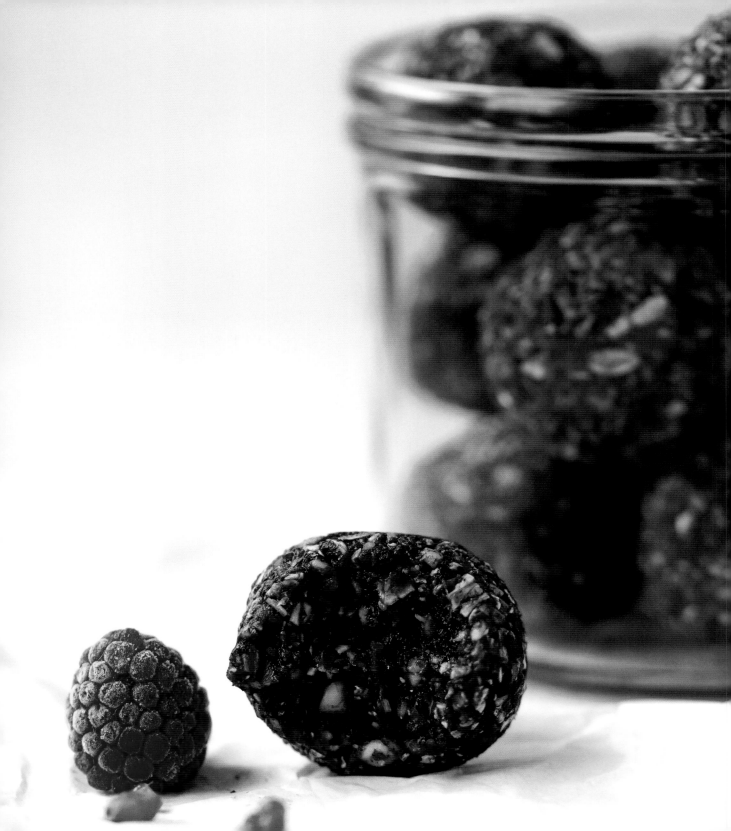

BERRY BALLS

HEALTHY SKIN

4 SERVINGS • Free radicals are unstable molecules that can cause cell damage, inflammation, and disease over time. One way to prevent these effects is by eating foods rich in antioxidants, such as açaí or maqui berry. Antioxidants work by stabilizing free radicals, thus helping prevent cell damage and its adverse effects. Maqui berry (*Aristotelia chilensis*) is an exotic, tiny, dark-purple berry that grows wild in South America. It's mainly harvested by the native Mapuche of Chile, an indigenous people who have used the leaves, stems, and berries medicinally for thousands of years. Today, maqui berry is marketed as a "superfruit" because of its high antioxidant content and potential health benefits.

1 cup oats

½ cup almonds

1 cup dates

½ cup frozen raspberries

1 teaspoon maqui powder, optional

1 teaspoon açaí powder

1 teaspoon tocos powder, optional

1 teaspoon vanilla extract, optional

BLEND all the ingredients together in a high-speed blender until sticky, then roll into 1½-inch balls.

STORE in a sealed container in the refrigerator for 3 to 5 days. Or freeze and store for about three months.

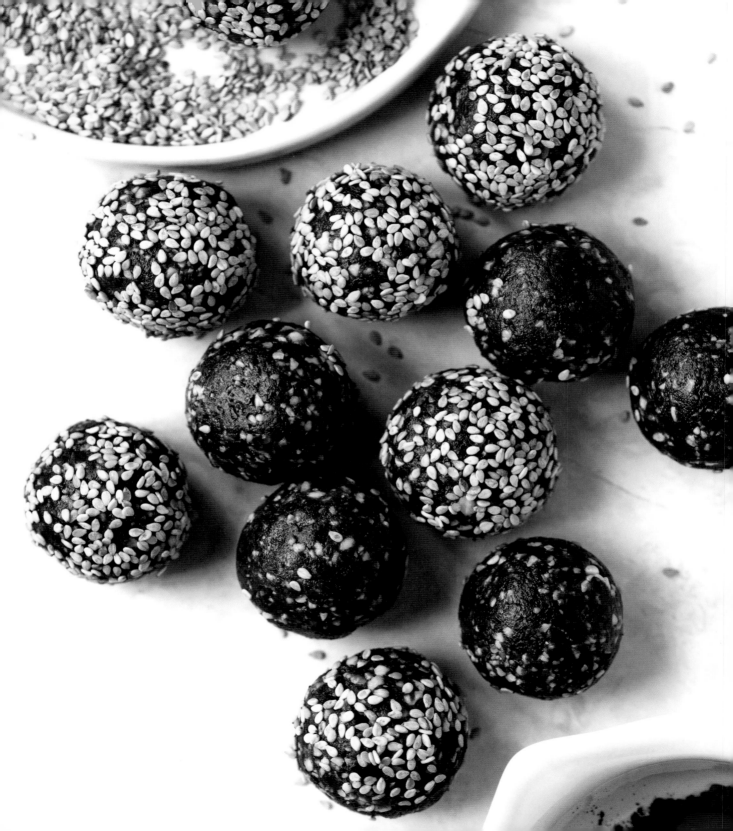

DATE TAHINI BALLS
ENERGY & IMMUNITY

4 SERVINGS • These balls were inspired by cuisines of the Middle East, where they know how out-of-this-world good dates and tahini are together. Dates are high in fiber, which is great for your digestive health and your microbiome, and potassium, magnesium, and manganese. They also contain the antioxidants flavonoids, carotenoids, and phenolic acid. Tahini and cashews are sources of healthy fats and protein.[3] We added superfoods guarana for energy and chaga for immune system support.

5 tablespoons tahini

¾ cup cashews

1 cup dates

1 tablespoon cacao nibs

½ teaspoon guarana powder, optional

½ teaspoon chaga powder, optional

Pinch of sea salt

⅓ cup sesame seeds, optional

BLEND the tahini, cashews, dates, cacao nibs, guarana and chaga, if using, and salt in a high-speed blender or food processor until sticky.

ROLL into 1½-inch balls in your hands. Roll the balls in the sesame seeds, if using.

STORE in an airtight container in the refrigerator for 3 to 5 days.

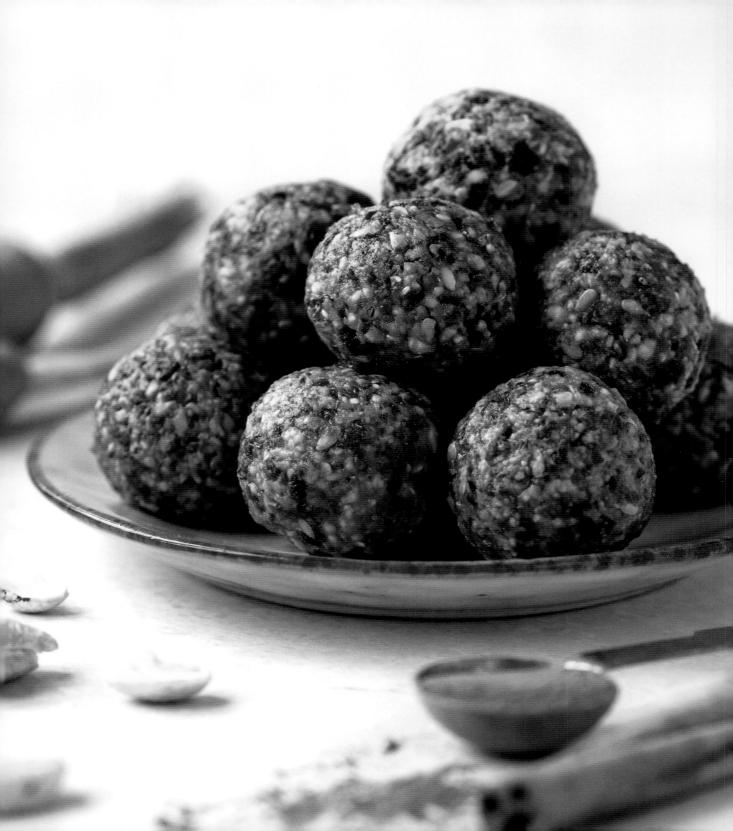

CARROT CAKE BALLS
PLANT PROTEIN & HEALTHY FATS

4 SERVINGS • It's not carrot cake but it's close! Flax and chia seeds are loaded with omega-3 fats, protein, and fiber. Omega-3s are important for brain health and heart health, while fiber supports your digestion. Tired of balls? You can also cut these in little squares—whatever shape you enjoy!

1 tablespoon flaxseeds	**1 cup cashews**
1 tablespoon chia seeds	**1 cup raisins**
⅓ cup grated carrot	**1 teaspoon cinnamon powder**
2 tablespoons pea protein powder	**1 teaspoon ginger powder**

PLACE all the ingredients together in a food processor or high-speed blender and process until sticky. Roll into balls.

STORE in a sealed container in the refrigerator for 3 to 5 days. Or freeze and store for about three months.

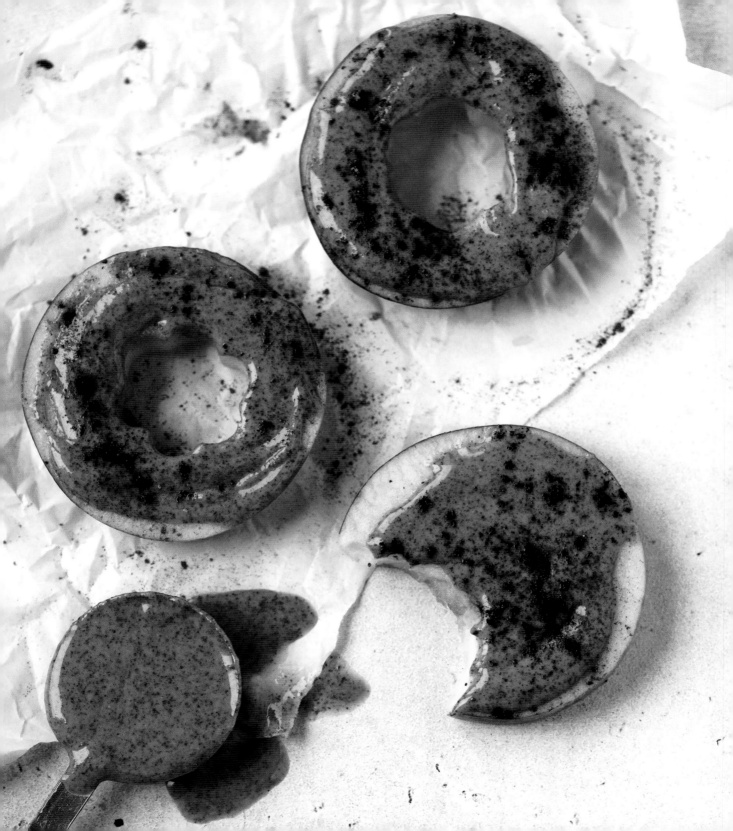

SUPER APPLE SLICES
HEALTHY SKIN & IMMUNITY

1 SERVING • This is my favorite "cheat" to get a superfood-rich snack into my day. It's like a dressed-up version of eating peanut butter from the jar. You can substitute bananas for the apples, and any fruity superfood powders are delicious on top. Just one teaspoon of açaí powder packs the same nutrition as a handful of berries.

1 apple

2 tablespoons almond butter

½ teaspoon baobab powder, optional

½ teaspoon acerola powder, optional

½ teaspoon açaí powder

½ teaspoon cinnamon powder

SLICE the apple.

SPREAD the almond butter on top.

MIX the superfood powders together in a small jar and sprinkle on top.

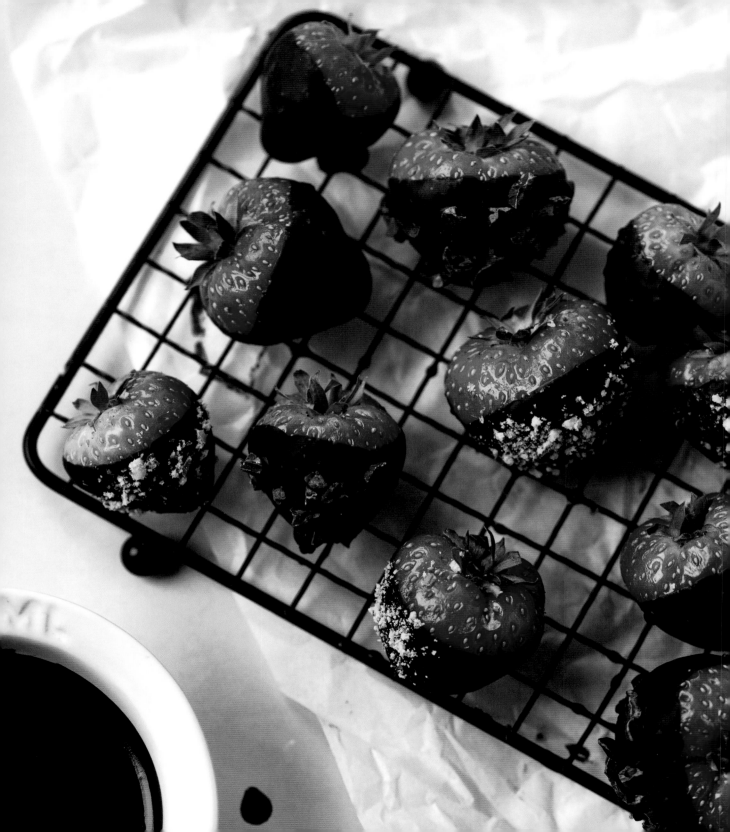

CHOCOLATE-DIPPED STRAWBERRIES
ENERGY & MOOD BOOSTER

2 SERVINGS · These aren't just for Valentine's Day! Antioxidant-boosting berries, long-lasting energy from guarana, plus cacao for a mood boost—how can you go wrong? If you prefer to skip the caffeine, choose a chaga or reishi mushroom powder to mix into the chocolate.

2 cups strawberries

3 tablespoons coconut oil

3 tablespoons cacao powder

1 tablespoon maple syrup

1 teaspoon chia seeds

½ teaspoon guarana powder, optional

Cacao nibs, optional

Crushed almonds, optional

WASH the strawberries and place them on a freezer-safe plate. Place in the freezer for 5 minutes.

IN a saucepan over low heat, stir together the coconut oil, cacao, maple syrup, chia seeds, and guarana, if using, until combined into a creamy, thick sauce, about 1 minute.

TAKE the strawberries from the freezer, dip them in the mixture, and put them back on the plate. Sprinkle cacao nibs and crushed almonds on top, if using. Put the plate back into the freezer for 10 minutes to set.

STORE in the fridge in an airtight container for 2 to 3 days.

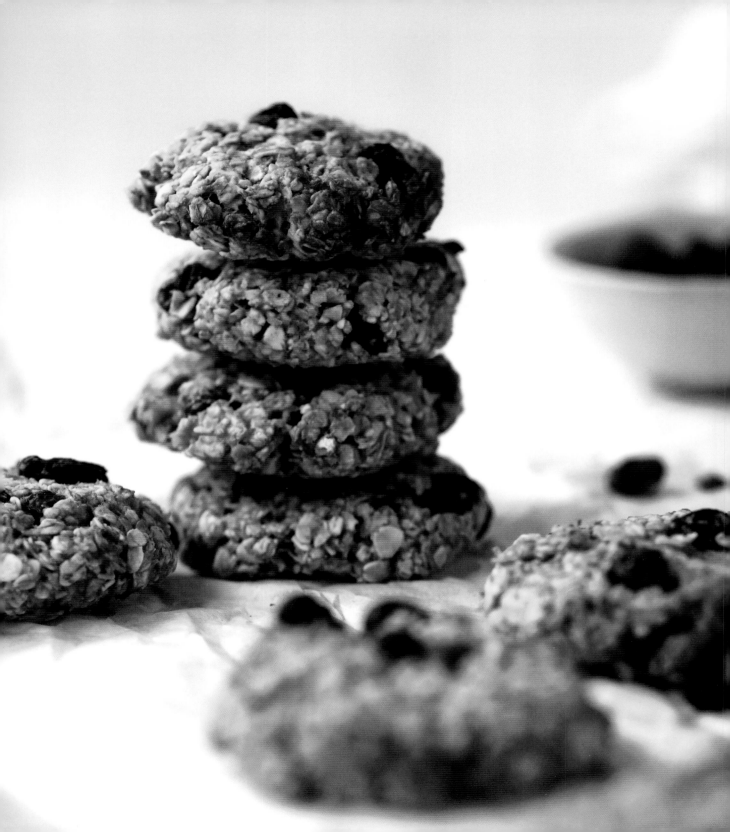

PROTEIN OAT COOKIES
PLANT PROTEIN & ANTI-INFLAMMATORY

4 SERVINGS • These cookies are easy to bake and chock-full of nutrition. Pea protein gives them a boost of extra protein, turmeric makes them anti-inflammatory and rich in antioxidants, and cinnamon means that unlike most cookies, these will actually support balanced blood sugar. The oats contain a ton of fiber to support your digestion.

2 cups quick oats

⅓ cup raisins

2 tablespoons pea protein powder

½ teaspoon turmeric powder, optional

1 teaspoon cinnamon powder

2 teaspoons tocos powder, optional

1 banana

3 tablespoons maple syrup

½ cup oat milk

PREHEAT the oven to 350°F. Line a baking sheet with parchment paper.

IN a medium-size bowl, combine the oats, raisins, pea protein, turmeric, if using, cinnamon, and tocos, if using.

IN a separate bowl mash the banana with a fork, and mix in the maple syrup and oat milk.

COMBINE the wet and dry ingredients and mix until you have a thick mixture, like cookie dough consistency. Add some water if needed.

SCOOP about 2 tablespoons of dough per cookie onto your baking sheet, making the cookies round and not too flat.

BAKE for 10 to 15 minutes until crispy on the outside and soft on the inside.

LET cool and enjoy! Store in a sealed container at room temperature for 3 to 4 days.

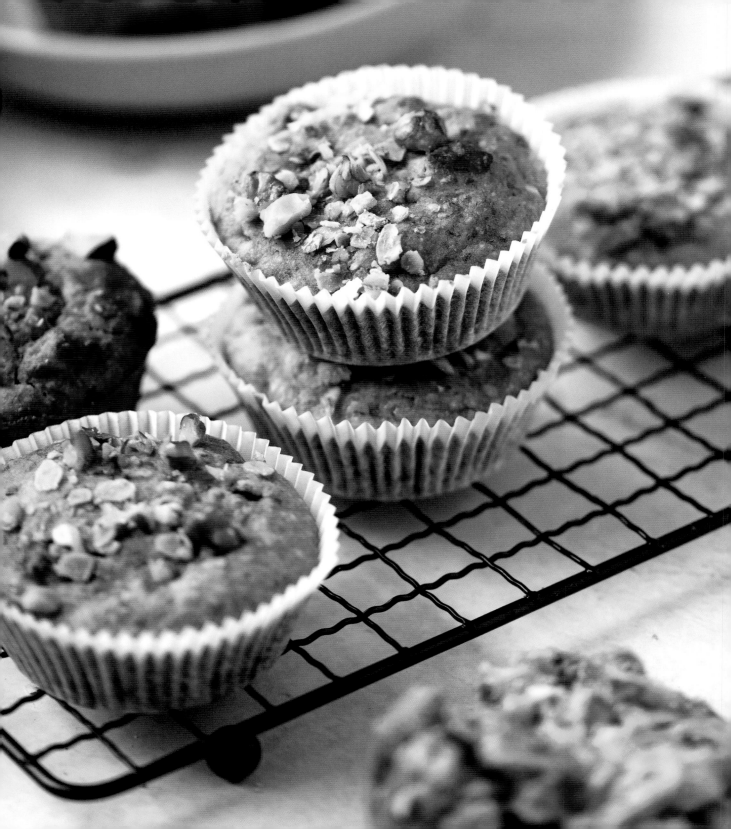

BANANA BREAD MUFFINS
HORMONE HEALTH & PLANT PROTEIN

MAKES 12 MUFFINS • If you love banana bread, you will love these muffins. You can swap the almond flour and oats with any type of flour you prefer. Over time, you can try experimenting with adding different superfoods for diverse health benefits and a variety of flavors. Turmeric and ginger, cacao and reishi, and açaí and dried cherries would make great alternatives. To make these extra pretty, top with walnuts and oats before baking.

3 ripe bananas, mashed

⅓ cup maple syrup

2 tablespoons flaxseeds

½ cup almond milk

⅓ cup melted coconut oil

1½ cups oat flour

¾ cup almond flour

1 teaspoon baking soda

4 teaspoons maca powder, optional

6 tablespoons pea protein powder

2 teaspoons cinnamon powder

2 tablespoons walnuts, chopped

2 tablespoons chia seeds

PREHEAT the oven to 375°F.

IN a large bowl, mix together the bananas, maple syrup, flaxseeds, almond milk, and coconut oil.

IN a separate bowl mix together the oat flour, almond flour, baking soda, maca, if using, pea protein powder, cinnamon, walnuts, and chia seeds.

COMBINE the wet and dry ingredients and stir together with a fork.

EVENLY divide batter among 12 muffin liners. Sprinkle tops with a few extra chopped walnuts to make them pretty.

BAKE for 18 to 25 minutes or until a tester inserted into the middle comes out clean or with just a few crumbs attached.

ALLOW muffins to cool in the pan for 5 to 10 minutes, then remove and transfer to a wire rack to finish cooling. Store in a sealed container at room temperature for up to 3 to 4 days.

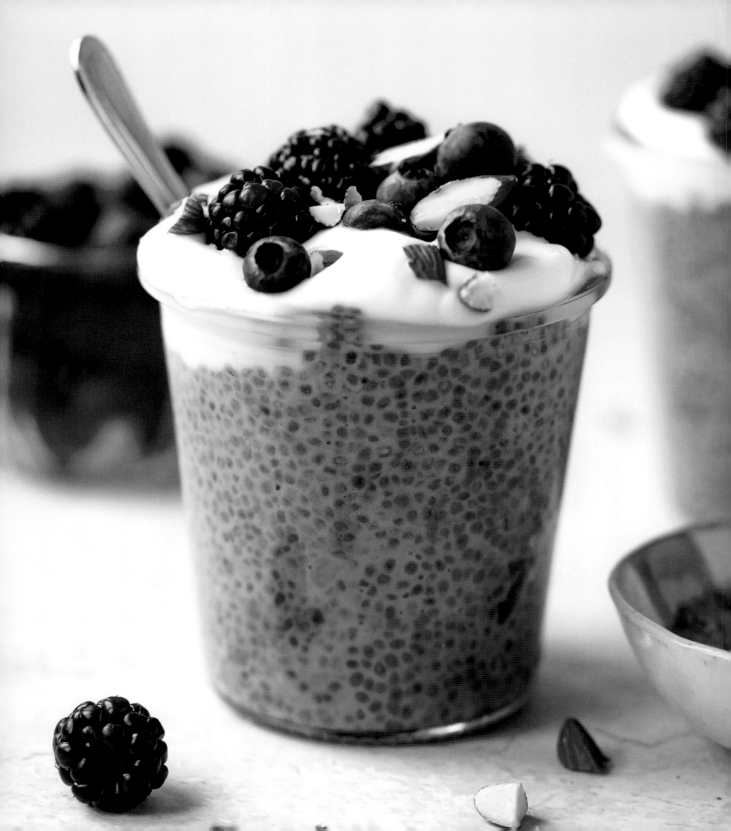

MATCHA CHIA PUDDING
ENERGY & HORMONE HEALTH

SERVES 2 • Chia seeds may be small, but they're incredibly rich in nutrients. A staple in the ancient Aztec and Maya diets, these seeds have been touted for their health benefits for centuries. The antioxidants, minerals, fiber, and omega-3 fatty acids in chia seeds may promote heart health, support strong bones, and improve blood sugar management. This recipe takes advantage of their gel-like consistency by mixing them with liquid and making chia pudding. Instead of energizing green tea matcha powder, you can use other superfood powder combinations like açaí and maqui, cacao and chaga, or turmeric and baobab. Unsweetened coconut, yogurt, berries, and chopped almonds make great garnishes.

½ banana

2 cups oat milk

½ cup chia seeds

2 tablespoons maple syrup

1 teaspoon matcha powder

1 teaspoon maca powder, optional

1 teaspoon vanilla extract, optional

CUT the banana into small half-moon slices.

IN a large bowl, mix together the banana slices, oat milk, chia seeds, maple syrup, matcha, and maca and vanilla extract, if using. Let the mixture stand for 5 minutes and stir again.

DIVIDE evenly between two 8–12 ounce jars. Close each jar with a lid and let them stand in the fridge for 1 or 2 hours or overnight.

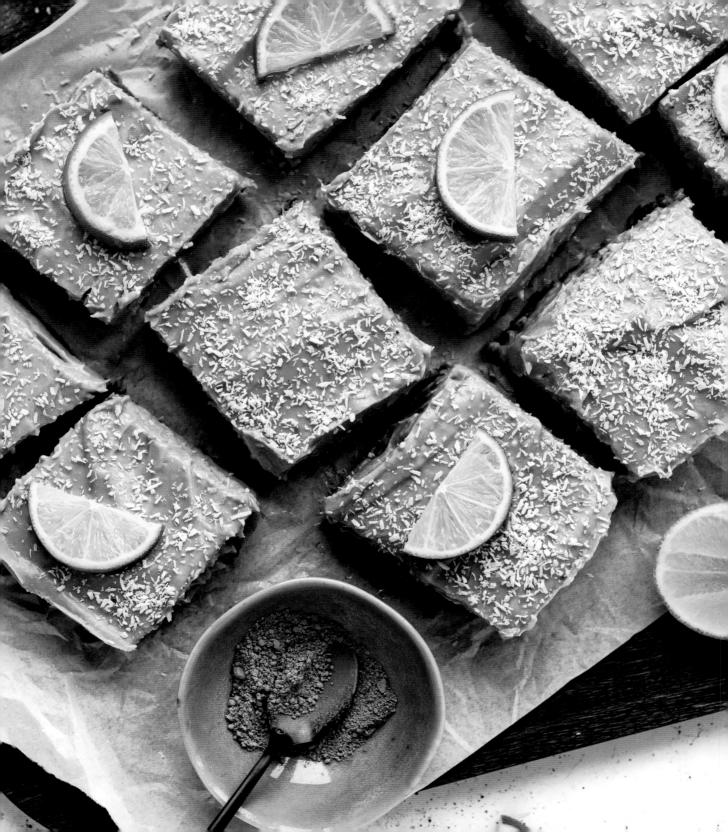

AVOCADO LIME SQUARES
ENERGY & IMMUNITY

SERVES 8 • The first time Kristel made this recipe with her sister, they couldn't believe how good it was and ate the whole thing in a day! The easy crust can be spiced up if you like by adding cacao or shredded coconut. You can also swap the pecans for cashews or almonds. You can use an oven dish, pie ring, or make them into cupcake shapes—it's up to you. This little energizing recipe is so indulgent you could totally serve it as birthday cake.

CRUST

1 cup pecans

1 cup dates

FILLING

½ cup coconut cream

4 ripe avocados, pitted

⅓ cup maple syrup

1 teaspoon matcha powder

1 teaspoon moringa powder, optional

2 teaspoon baobab powder, optional

½ cup lime juice (from 3 or 4 limes)

1 tablespoon lime zest

STORE a can of coconut milk in the fridge overnight and scoop only the cream from the top.

IN a high-speed blender or food processor combine the pecans and dates together and blend until you've got a sticky mixture.

LINE an 8x8-inch freezer-safe dish with parchment paper and add the sticky mixture to the bottom and sides of the dish. Freeze for 30 minutes.

MIX all the filling ingredients together in a high-speed blender and process until smooth. Mixture will be thick. Pour the filling into the crust. Return the pie to the freezer for 3 or 4 hours then cut into squares and enjoy.

STORE the bars in the fridge in an airtight container for 3 to 4 days.

HOW TO MAKE PLANT MILK

You can buy plant milks at most groceries these days, but we still love the taste and fresh factor of making our own—and it's much simpler than you may realize. Following the steps below will create 3 to 4 servings of plant milk.

① CHOOSE YOUR BASE

Mix and match 1 cup from the following ingredients: almonds, brazil nuts, cashews, hazelnuts, macadamia, pecans, pistachios, walnuts, oats, nut butter, or hemp seeds.

② ADD TO THE BLENDER

Add 3½ cups of water. Add 1 pitted date or 2 teaspoons maple syrup to sweeten, a pinch of sea salt to taste, and any desired superfoods for extra benefits.

③ BLEND

It works best with a high-speed blender. Blend for 1 or 2 minutes until smooth and creamy.

④ STRAIN (IF NECESSARY)

This step is only necessary if you're using a nut that has skin, for example, almonds, brazil nuts, or hazelnuts. You do not have to strain the nut milk of cashews, macadamias, and walnuts. You need a super-fine strainer like a nut milk bag.

⑤ STORE

Pour your milk in a pitcher and store in the fridge for up to 3 to 5 days.

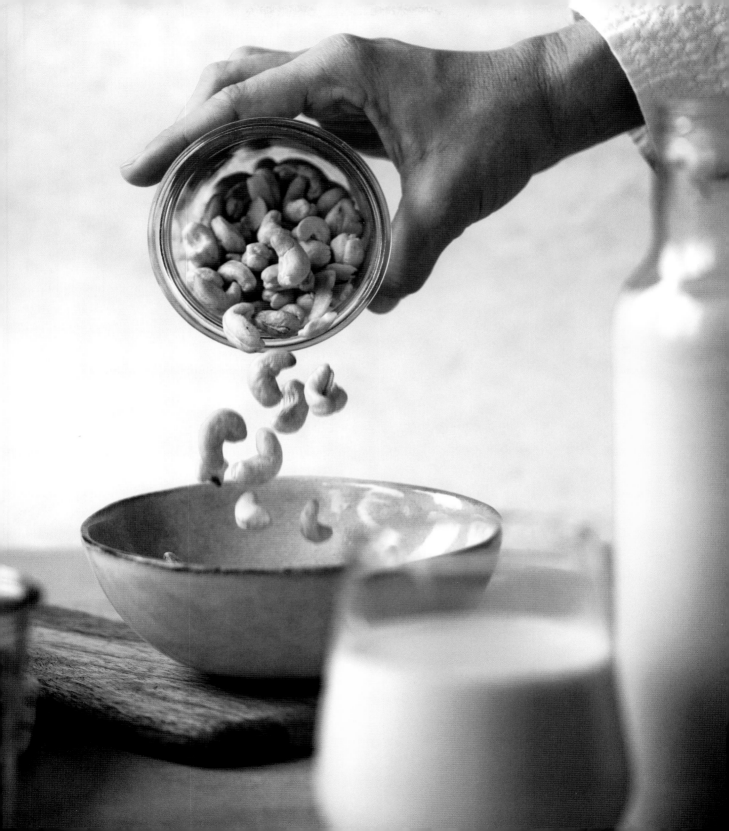

HOW TO MAKE POWER BALLS

Loaded with nutrients to keep you focused and going strong no matter what life throws at you, power balls are a great, healthy snack option. The best part: You need only a few ingredients, a food processor or blender, and five minutes. This is the perfect snack to prep ahead of time—your friends and family will love them.

① CHOOSE YOUR BASE

Mix and match 1 cup from the following ingredients: almonds, brazil nuts, cashews, hazelnuts, macadamias, pecans, pistachios, walnuts, coconut flakes, cacao nibs, or oats.

② SWEET & STICKY

Mix and match 1 cup from dried fruits like dates, raisins, figs, apricots, cherries, cranberries, goji, mango, pineapple, or banana. Plus butters like almond, peanut, cashew, or tahini, and sweeteners such as maple syrup and dates.

③ ADD YOUR SUPERFOODS

Add 3 teaspoons of your favorite superfoods for an extra health boost and more flavor. Choose superfoods such as açaí, maqui, cacao, wheatgrass, maca, shatavari, spirulina, chaga, reishi, ginger, turmeric, baobab, chia seeds, acerola, etc.

④ EXTRA FLAVOR

Add a pinch of sea salt, cinnamon, cardamom, chai, nutmeg, or chili powder.

⑤ BLEND

Use a food processor or blender to mix everything together. You might need to scrape the sides in between. Blend long enough for the oils to release from the nuts; often this can take at least 2 or 3 minutes. When no longer sticky, add some melted coconut oil, maple syrup, or nut butter. Have fun finding your favorite combination.

⑥ DECORATE (OPTIONAL)

Roll into bite-size balls. If desired, you can roll the sticky balls into a decoration or dusting to give them a cool look and more exciting texture. Also if you get tired of balls, you can mold this snack in any shape you like, such as squares or bars. Store in a sealed container in the fridge for 3 to 5 days. You can also freeze them if you'd like to keep them longer. Decorations to use are shredded coconut, chia seeds, broken nuts, sesame seeds, or superfood powders.

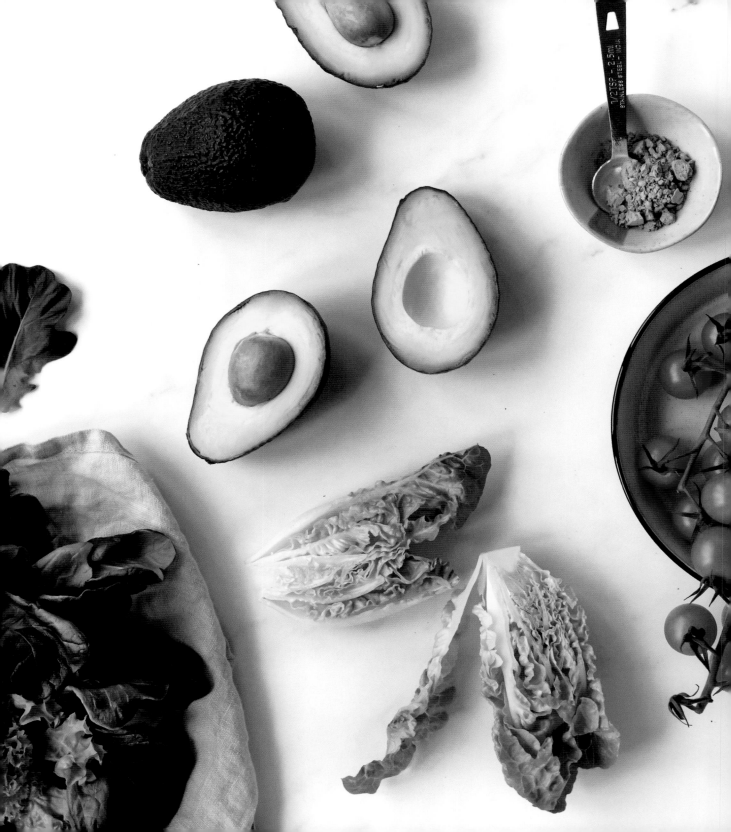

DIGEST

EASY NOURISHING LUNCHES

Did you know that eating while stressed can actually reduce the absorption of vital nutrients? Not to mention that stress slows down digestion. We wanted to give you plenty of filling, nutritious lunch recipes that are quick to make and include lots of nutrient-rich superfoods.

We tend to focus on eating more raw foods at lunch so that we feel full but light and not tired. In this chapter, you'll find lots of greens and salads bursting with colorful veggies, along with a carb and/or protein so that you stay full and satisfied for hours. Eating raw fresh veggies makes you feel vibrant. But when you're craving something warm, we've also got plenty of soups and some creative toasts for you too. You can also add superfoods to your savory meals—they are especially easy to add to homemade dressings and dips.

Kristel likes to prep and cook veggies ahead of time so she can throw lunch together quickly (and spend more time decompressing and less time cooking). If you are super busy, eat your leftovers from dinner with a small fresh salad and veggies for lunch.

Try not to eat in front of your laptop. Being present while you eat helps you stay in the moment and actually enjoy what you're eating. And paying attention while we are eating allows us to feel the fullness of our stomachs, which helps us to easily eat the right amount of food.

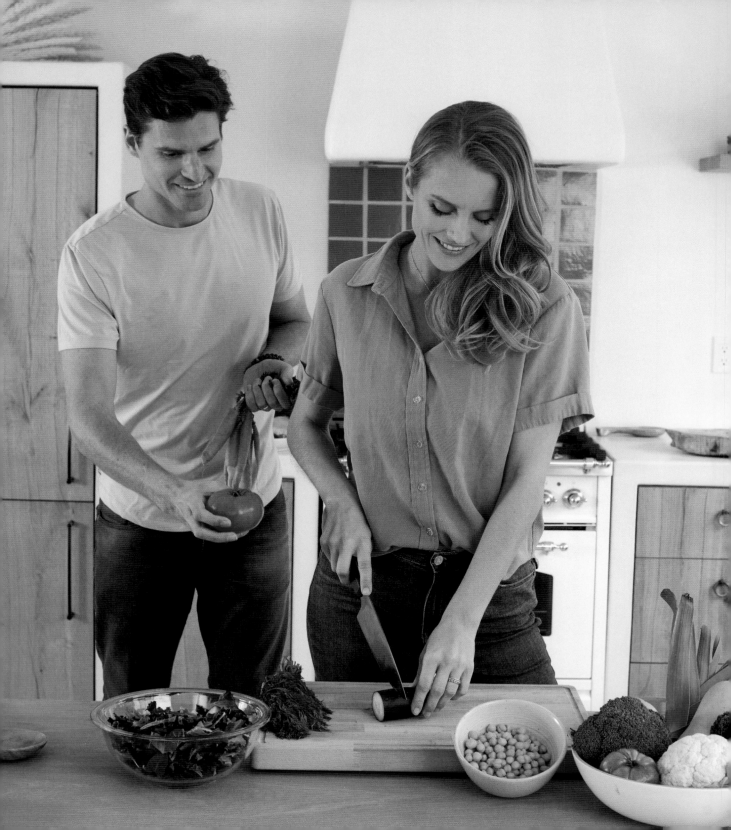

EASY GREEN SALAD
IMMUNITY & HEALTHY FATS

SERVES 1 • This is one of our favorite go-to salads—we simply can't get enough of it. We're also all about making easy delicious dressings at home. Use nut and seed butters as a base plus something vinegary or acidic—in this case lemon juice—and your favorite herbs, spices, and superfood powders and you can make delicious combinations that you simply stir together with a fork and enjoy in less than three minutes. We love adding extra crunch to salads with crushed flaxseed crackers on top. Buy your favorite flaxseed crackers or make your own (see page 189).

½ medium-size head of romaine lettuce, washed and chopped

1 tomato, chopped

½ cucumber, cubed

2 tablespoons capers

2 scallion stalks, sliced

½ avocado, pitted and sliced

½ can (7.5 ounces) white beans, about ¾ cup, drained and rinsed

½ cup crushed flaxseed crackers, optional

DRESSING

2 tablespoons tahini

Juice of ½ lemon

1 teaspoon baobab powder, optional

½ teaspoon garlic powder

Sea salt and pepper to taste

COMBINE the veggies, avocado, and beans in a shallow bowl.

COMBINE all the dressing ingredients in a glass jar or bowl and stir with a fork for about a minute until smooth and creamy.

POUR dressing on top and toss gently.

TOP it off with crushed flaxseed crackers, if you desire, for extra crunch.

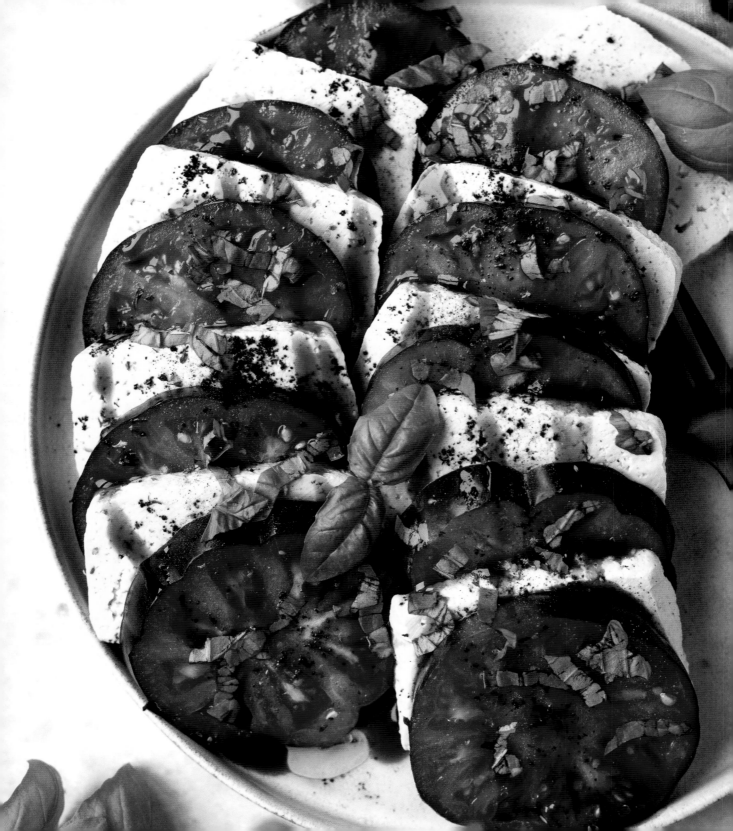

TOMATO TOFU PLATTER
HEALTHY SKIN & PLANT PROTEIN

SERVES 1 • This is a nourishing twist on your classic tomato mozzarella platter. You can substitute vegan mozzarella for the tofu if it's available in your area. We like to use heirloom tomatoes, which are varieties that have been grown without crossbreeding for forty or more years. Heirlooms usually haven't been hybridized for qualities like shelf life, color, and uniform appearance. They are often "ugly" with deep cracks and bumps, but don't be turned off by their looks—they often taste better! If you're new to tofu and aren't sure you'll like the taste, you can marinate it in the dressing for 15 minutes or overnight to give it more flavor. Simply make your dressing, marinate the tofu overnight, and then layer the tofu over your tomato slices.

2 large tomatoes, heirloom variety
if possible

6 ounces extra-firm tofu

½ cup fresh basil

3 tablespoons balsamic vinegar

1 tablespoon olive oil, optional

1 teaspoon açaí powder, optional

Sea salt and pepper to taste

1 teaspoon dried Italian herbs

SLICE the tomatoes and spread them out in a single layer on a big plate.

PRESS and drain the tofu, wrap it in a clean kitchen towel, and put it on a large plate. Place something heavy—another plate works or a frying pan or a cookbook—and press to squeeze out moisture. Slice the tofu about ¼ inch thick and layer one slice on each of the tomato slices.

CHOP the basil in thin slices and sprinkle over the top.

IN a small bowl combine the balsamic vinegar, olive oil, açaí, if using, salt and pepper, and Italian herbs, and stir until well blended. Drizzle over the tomato and tofu slices.

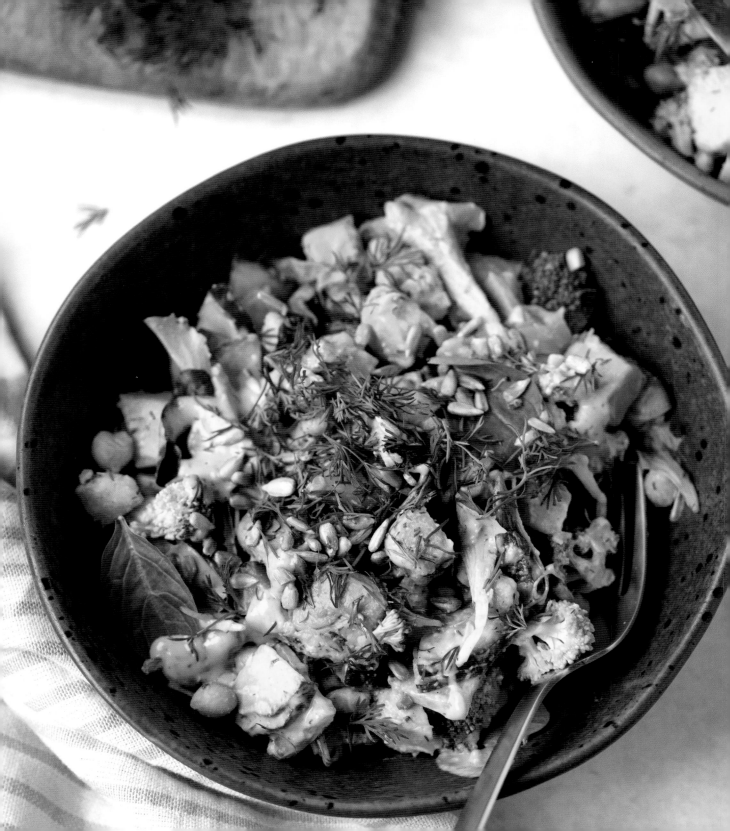

POTATO DILL SALAD
IMMUNITY & ANTI-INFLAMMATORY

SERVES 1 • We love adding fresh herbs to any salad because they are loaded with micronutrients and add a pop of flavor. Think basil, parsley, cilantro, chives, mint, thyme, and in this recipe, dill! Dill is a medicinal herb that has been used for more than 2,000 years. Rich in antioxidants and a good source of vitamin C, magnesium, and vitamin A, it combines beautifully with the mustard in this dressing. Go ahead and make a double batch of dressing for dipping crackers and veggies—it stores well for up to 5 days in the fridge. Garnish with chopped dill and sunflower seeds.

1 purple sweet potato, washed and cubed

3 cups salad greens of your choice

¼ cucumber, chopped

½ avocado, pitted and cubed

½ can (7.5 ounces) chickpeas, about ¾ cup, drained and rinsed

1 cup broccoli florets

¼ cup fresh dill, chopped, optional

DRESSING

2 teaspoon dried dill

3 tablespoons ground mustard

1 tablespoon tahini

½ teaspoon turmeric powder

Sea salt and pepper to taste

BRING a pot of water to boil over high heat. Add the potato cubes and cook until soft, 15 to 20 minutes. Drain and set aside.

IN a large bowl, combine potatoes, salad greens, cucumber, avocado, chickpeas, broccoli, and fresh dill, if using.

TO make the dressing, combine the dried dill, mustard, tahini, turmeric, and salt and pepper in a glass jar or a bowl, and stir with a fork until smooth, adding water to thin as needed.

POUR the dressing over the salad and toss gently to combine. Enjoy!

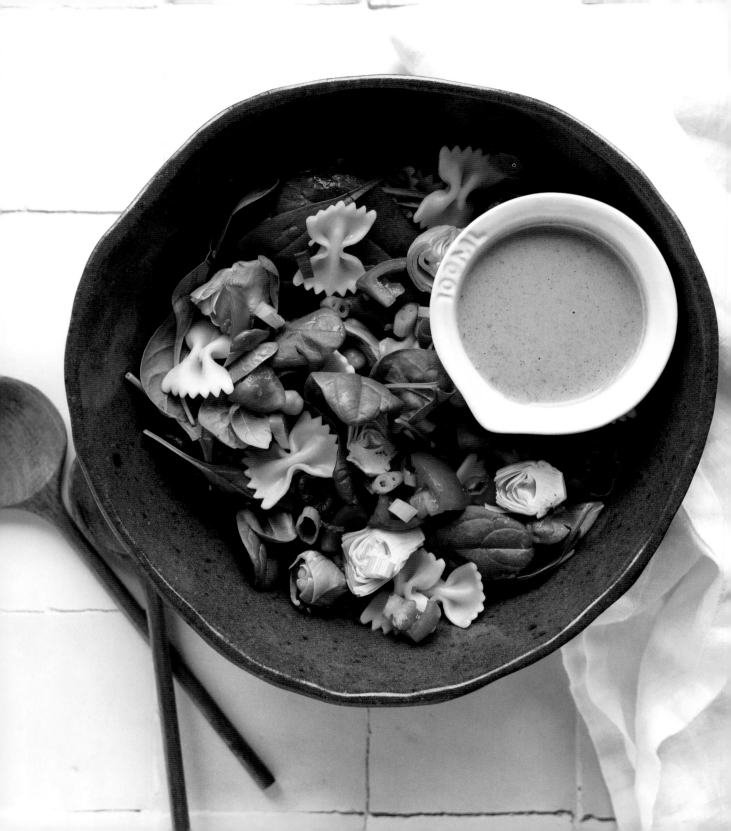

ITALIAN-INSPIRED ANTIPASTO SALAD
IMMUNITY & PLANT PROTEIN

SERVES 1 • Adding olives, artichokes, and other Italian antipasti like capers are a great way to add more flavor to your salads. That's what we've done here in this salad, inspired by the original. Combined with fresh leafy greens and veggies you have a delicious salad going for you. If, like us, you love adding a carb to your salad to make it more filling, use pasta. Chickpeas add more plant protein and fiber. This salad has all the familiar flavors of a traditional antipasto, with a healthy twist!!

Leftover pasta or 1 cup gluten-free pasta, cooked according to package directions

1 scallion, chopped

½ red bell pepper, diced

1 tomato, diced

3 canned artichokes, drained and chopped

¼ cup pitted olives, halved

2 cups baby spinach

¼ cup canned chickpeas, drained and rinsed

4 stalks fresh basil

DRESSING

2 tablespoons tahini

2 tablespoons balsamic vinegar

Sea salt and pepper to taste

1 teaspoon dried Italian herbs

COMBINE pasta, scallion, pepper, tomato, artichokes, olives, spinach, chickpeas, and basil in a big bowl.

TO make the dressing, place tahini, vinegar, salt and pepper, and Italian herbs in a jar and stir with a fork to combine, adding water to thin as needed.

ADD dressing to your salad and toss to coat.

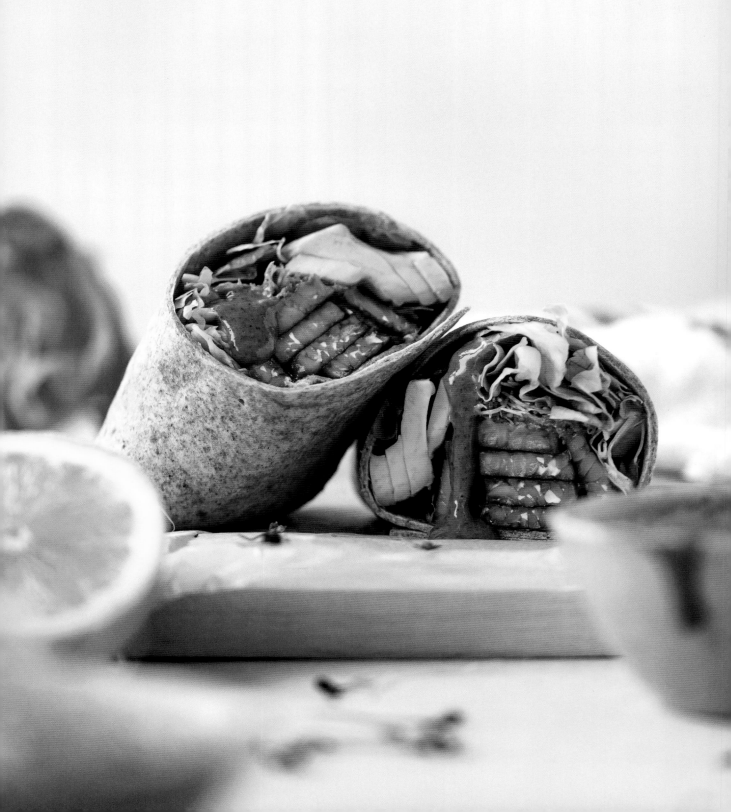

TEMPEH WRAP
IMMUNITY & PLANT PROTEIN

SERVES 1 • While we love salads for lunch, sometimes you need a bit more variety. An easy trick is put your salad in a wrap. This gives you the mouthfeel of a sandwich with a healthy dose of raw veggies to fuel you through the remainder of your day. Tempeh gives this wrap a good meaty bite; combined with the barbecue-inspired dipping sauce, this is a filling and delicious lunch. The baobab powder gives it some freshness and an extra boost of vitamin C. Feel free to switch up the veggies—sliced red bell pepper, cucumber, tomato, and romaine lettuce all work well.

1 tablespoon coconut oil

1 cup tempeh, sliced

1 tablespoon tamari

Pepper, to taste

SAUCE

2 tablespoons almond butter

Juice of ½ lemon

1 teaspoon baobab powder, optional

1 tablespoon tamari sauce

2 cups alfalfa sprouts

½ avocado, sliced

Gluten-free wrap from buckwheat, coconut, corn, or almond

¼ teaspoon chili powder

½ teaspoon garlic powder

Sea salt and pepper to taste

IN a wok or large skillet on high heat, add the coconut oil and then the tempeh. Stir for 5 minutes. Add the tamari and pepper. Stir for another 5 minutes until the tempeh is crispy.

STIR all the sauce ingredients together in a glass with a fork until creamy and smooth. Add water to find the right consistency.

MAKE your wrap: Fill each wrap with the tempeh mixture, and top with the sprouts, avocado, and sauce.

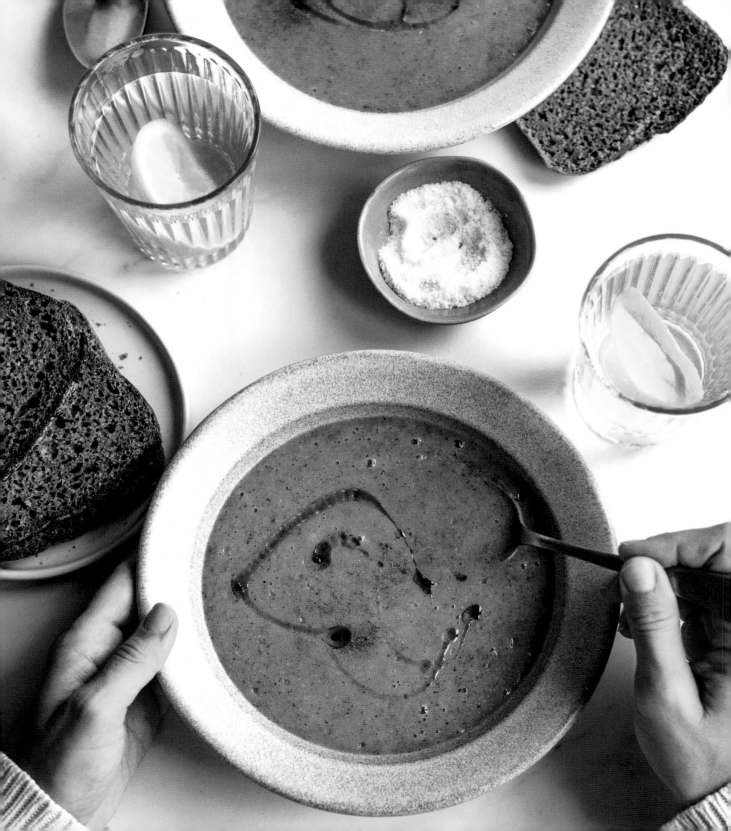

GREEN SOUP
DETOX & IMMUNITY

SERVES 2 • A good green soup is simply good for the soul and this is by far one of our favorites. It's perfect on colder days when you don't feel like eating raw veggies but still want to get your greens in! Ginger boosts your immunity, moringa contains all essential vitamins and minerals, broccoli is a nutritional powerhouse full of vitamins, minerals, fiber, and antioxidants. You can hide any other green superfoods in this soup so don't be shy!

4 medium potatoes, cubed

1 onion, diced

1 inch fresh ginger root, chopped

1 zucchini, diced

½ head broccoli, chopped

2 teaspoons moringa powder, optional

½ teaspoon garlic powder

Sea salt and pepper to taste

ADD the potatoes, onions, and ginger to 5 cups of boiling water and cook for 15 minutes.

AFTER 15 minutes, add the zucchini and broccoli and boil for 5 to 10 more minutes.

TURN the heat off and add the moringa, garlic powder, and salt and pepper and stir to combine.

LADLE soup in batches into a high-speed blender or use an immersion blender to puree. Add more water if it gets too thick. Serve hot.

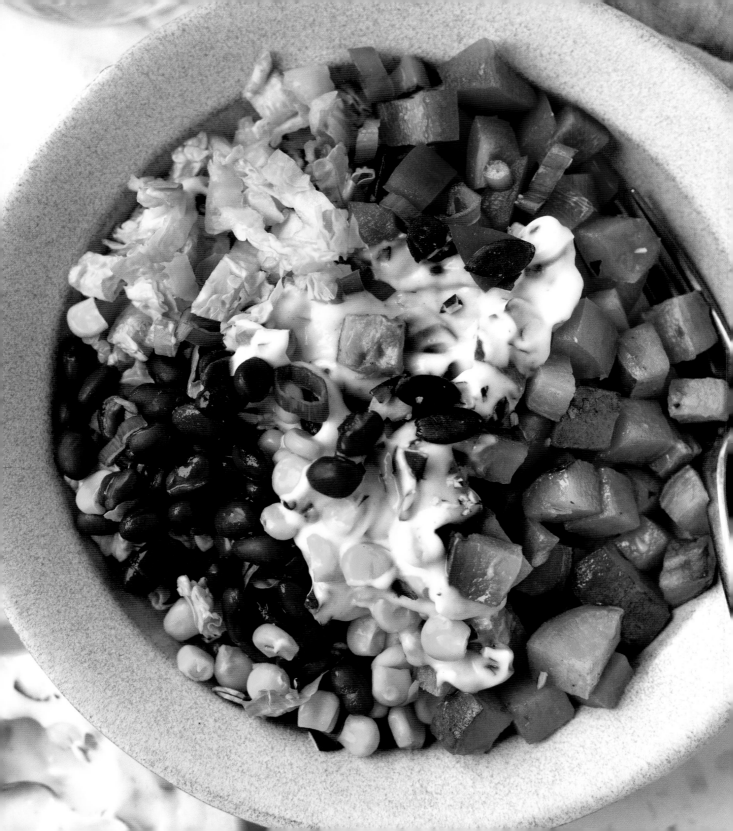

MEXICAN-STYLE BOWL
IMMUNITY & PLANT PROTEIN

SERVES 1 • This bowl was inspired by our favorite Mexican dishes and combines corn, tomatoes, and black beans with a touch of lime. The creamy dressing on this bowl combines acerola cherry powder, which is one of the highest natural sources of vitamin C, with the cleansing power of cilantro. It's a true health booster hidden in a refreshing, yummy dressing! Did you know that red bell pepper also contains a lot of vitamin C—a medium-size red bell pepper provides 169 percent of the Reference Daily Intake (RDI) for vitamin C? To make this bowl even more filling, add roasted or cooked sweet potato.

½ cup fresh or frozen corn

1 tomato, diced

½ can (7.5 ounces) black beans, about ¾ cup, drained and rinsed

½ head romaine lettuce, chopped

½ red bell pepper, diced

1 scallion, sliced

1 cup cubed sweet potato, roasted or boiled, optional

2 tablespoons pumpkin seeds

DRESSING

½ cup plain, unsweetened almond or soy yogurt

Zest and juice of 1 lime

⅓ cup fresh cilantro, chopped

½ teaspoon garlic powder

½ teaspoon chili powder

½ teaspoon acerola powder, optional

½ teaspoon sea salt

COMBINE corn, tomato, black beans, lettuce, bell pepper, scallions, sweet potatoes, if using, and pumpkin seeds in a large bowl.

TO make the dressing, combine all ingredients in a glass jar or bowl and stir to combine.

ADD the dressing to salad and toss to combine. Enjoy!

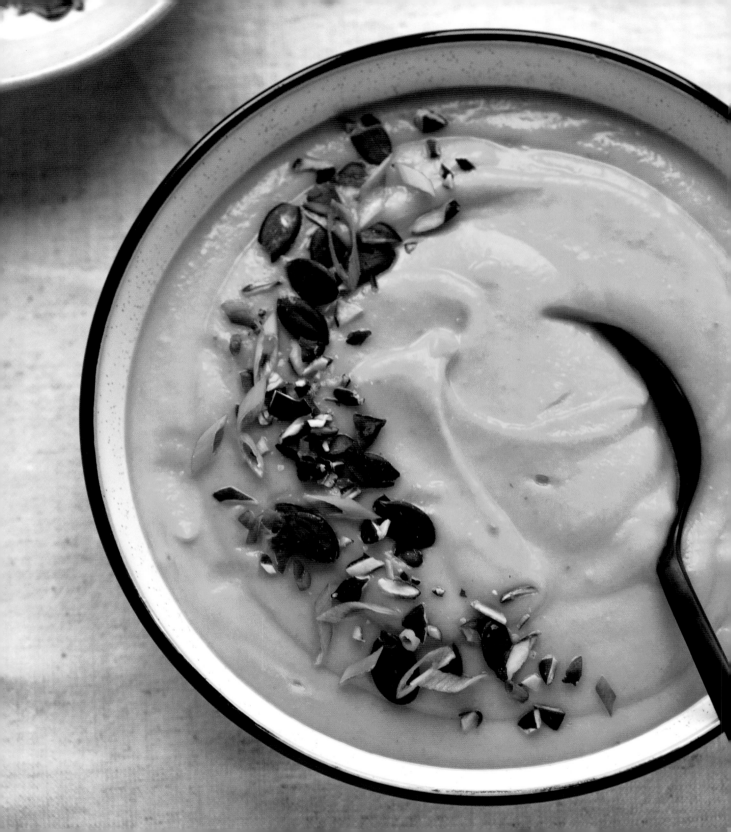

PUMPKIN SOUP
IMMUNITY & ANTI-INFLAMMATORY

SERVES 2 • Any pumpkin or squash works in this recipe so pick your favorite—whether it's butternut, winter squash, delicata, classic, or jack-o'-lantern orange. Simply boil raw pumpkin until tender, or use leftover roasted pumpkin. We combine the sweet pumpkin with warming Indian spices like turmeric, ginger, and tulsi—true superfoods that also add a little spice. Roasted veggies are the perfect base for any soup. In fact, Kristel's trick to make a quick soup in 5 minutes without cooking is to blend your leftover roasted veggies with spices, some coconut cream or nut butter for creaminess, and hot boiling water—that's it. Hacks like these make healthy eating every day sustainable, no matter how busy life gets. Garnish with pumpkin seeds and scallions.

1 small pumpkin, about 2 pounds

1 onion, diced

4 garlic cloves, minced

1 cup canned coconut milk

2 teaspoons curry powder

1 teaspoon ginger powder

1 teaspoon turmeric powder

1 teaspoon tulsi powder, optional

Sea salt and pepper to taste

LEAVING the skin on, slice open your pumpkin, scoop out the seeds, and cut it into 1-inch cubes. You should have 8 cups of pumpkin cubes.

IN a large pot, combine the pumpkin, onion, garlic, coconut milk, curry, ginger, turmeric, tulsi, and salt and pepper with six cups of water and bring to a boil.

TURN down to a simmer and cook for 20 to 30 minutes or until the pumpkin is soft and breaks up easily.

LADLE the soup into a high-speed blender and puree until smooth. Or use an immersion blender. Add hot water if it gets too thick. Serve immediately.

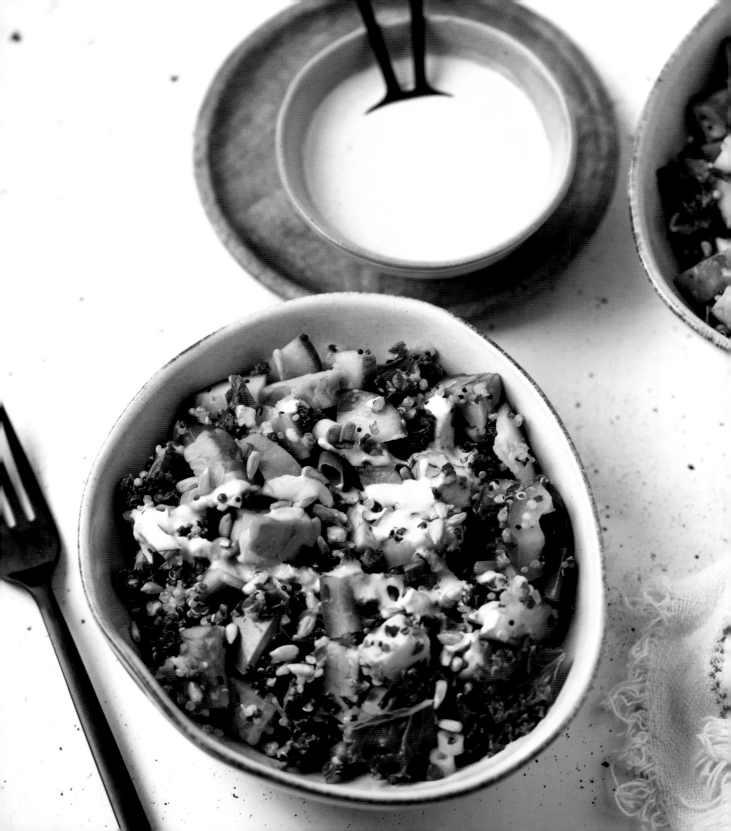

QUINOA TEMPEH SALAD
DETOX & IMMUNITY

SERVES 1 • This salad is all about the dressing—creamy cashew butter is the base, nutritional yeast gives it a cheesy umami flavor, and spirulina supports your body with tons of nutrients and detoxification. With fresh veggies, tempeh, and quinoa for protein and fiber, this salad pretty much has it all. Quinoa is a nutrient-packed grain that was initially cultivated more than 5,000 years ago and is traced to the Inca civilization of South America.

SALAD

¼ cup quinoa

1 cup cubed tempeh

1 teaspoon tamari

2 cups kale, destemmed and chopped

¼ cucumber, diced

½ green bell pepper, seeded and diced

½ avocado, pitted and cubed

2 tablespoons capers

1 scallion, sliced

1 tablespoon sunflower seeds, optional

1 teaspoon kelp or nori flakes, optional

DRESSING

3 tablespoons cashew butter

½ teaspoon spirulina powder, optional

1 teaspoon garlic powder

1 tablespoon nutritional yeast

Sea salt and pepper to taste

COOK the quinoa according to package directions.

IN a small ceramic-coated stir-fry pan, cook the tempeh with the tamari sauce over medium heat for 5 minutes, until warm and combined.

COMBINE the quinoa, tempeh, kale, cucumber, bell pepper, avocado, capers, scallion, and sunflower seeds and kelp, if using, in a large bowl.

TO make dressing, combine all ingredients in a small glass jar or bowl and stir together with a fork until creamy, adding water if necessary to thin.

POUR dressing over salad and toss to combine. Enjoy!

HEALTHY SPROUT SALAD
IMMUNITY & HEALTHY FATS

SERVES 1 • In most stores you can buy a variety of sprouts and microgreens like broccoli, clover, alfalfa, and mung bean sprouts. Grab what you can find and combine it all for a powerfully nutritious salad base. Sprouts are raw and live foods that are packed with nutrients. If you're curious about growing your own sprouts, the easiest to start with are mung beans, which sprout within 2 or 3 days. You don't need any fancy kitchen tools. You can get a stackable sprouter kit for around $15. Spread out the mung beans on the tray and rinse them with water 2 or 3 times a day for 2 or 3 days until they are sprouted—they'll be nice and crunchy.

1 cup mung bean sprouts

2 cups alfalfa, clover, or broccoli sprouts

¼ cucumber, diced

½ red bell pepper, seeded and diced

4 tablespoons sauerkraut

2 tablespoons sliced olives

½ can (7.5 ounces) kidney beans, about ¾ cup, drained and rinsed

½ avocado, pitted and diced

½ cup fresh parsley, finely chopped

1½ cups flaxseed crackers—store-bought or make your own (see page 189)

DRESSING

2 tablespoons tahini

Juice of ½ lemon

1 teaspoon baobab powder, optional

½ teaspoon garlic powder

Sea salt and pepper, to taste

COMBINE the sprouts, cucumber, bell pepper, sauerkraut, olives, kidney beans, avocado, and parsley in a large bowl.

TO make dressing, combine all the ingredients in a jar and stir with a fork for about a minute, until smooth and creamy, adding water if necessary to thin.

DRIZZLE the dressing on the salad and top with crumbled flaxseed crackers for extra crunch.

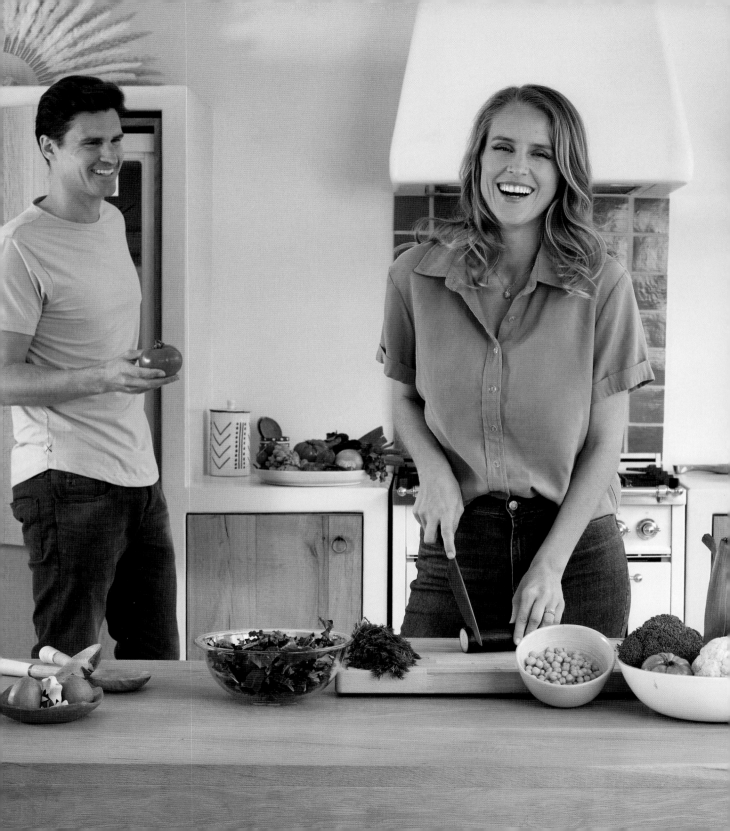

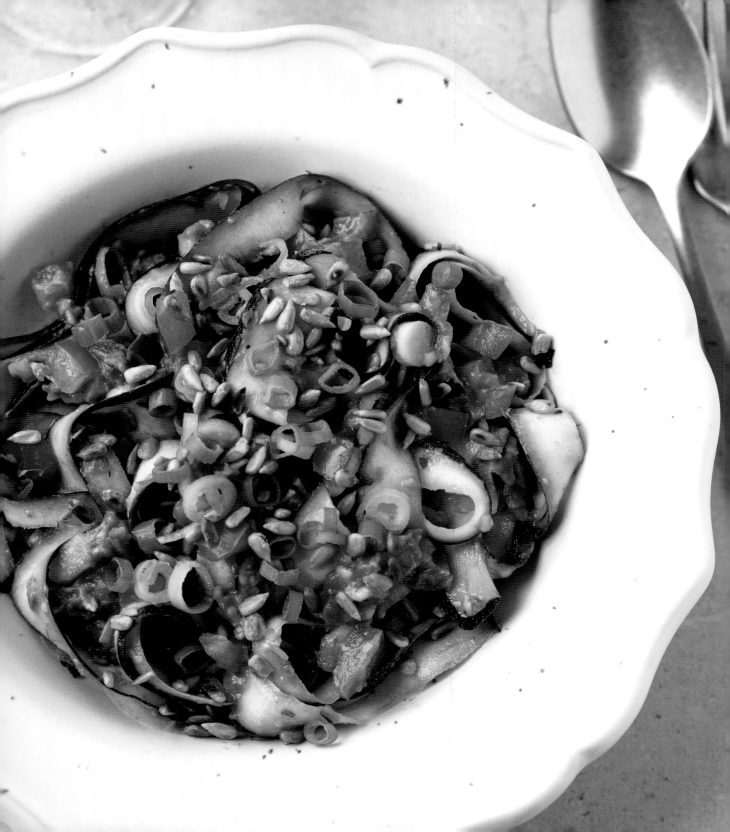

ZUCCHINI PASTA SALAD
DETOX & IMMUNITY

SERVES 1 • Zucchini pasta combined with fresh tomatoes, basil, olives, and green onion—this simple salad is, oh, so good. The sauce is super creamy thanks to the avocado and has a nice strong flavor because of the sun-dried tomatoes, so you can't detect the added superfoods. We like wheatgrass, but feel free to experiment. You can use any Italian herb blend—premixed blends are super easy. Spiralize the zucchini for a spaghetti-like base or simply use a peeler for a wider, flat tagliatelle-like feel. Garnish with sunflower seeds and scallions.

1 zucchini

1 tomato, diced

½ cup fresh basil, chopped

DRESSING

½ avocado

5 sun-dried tomatoes

1 teaspoon dried Italian herbs

10 kalamata olives, pitted and halved, optional

2 tablespoons sunflower seeds, optional

1 scallion, sliced

½ teaspoon wheatgrass powder, optional

Sea salt and pepper to taste

SLICE the zucchini in half lengthwise and use a peeler or spiralizer to make thick slices or thin "zoodles."

COMBINE zucchini, diced tomato, basil, and olives in a medium-size bowl.

TO make dressing, process all the ingredients in a blender or with a hand mixer, adding water to thin as needed, until you have a thick but pourable creamy sauce.

TOP the salad with the dressing and sunflower seeds and scallions, if desired.

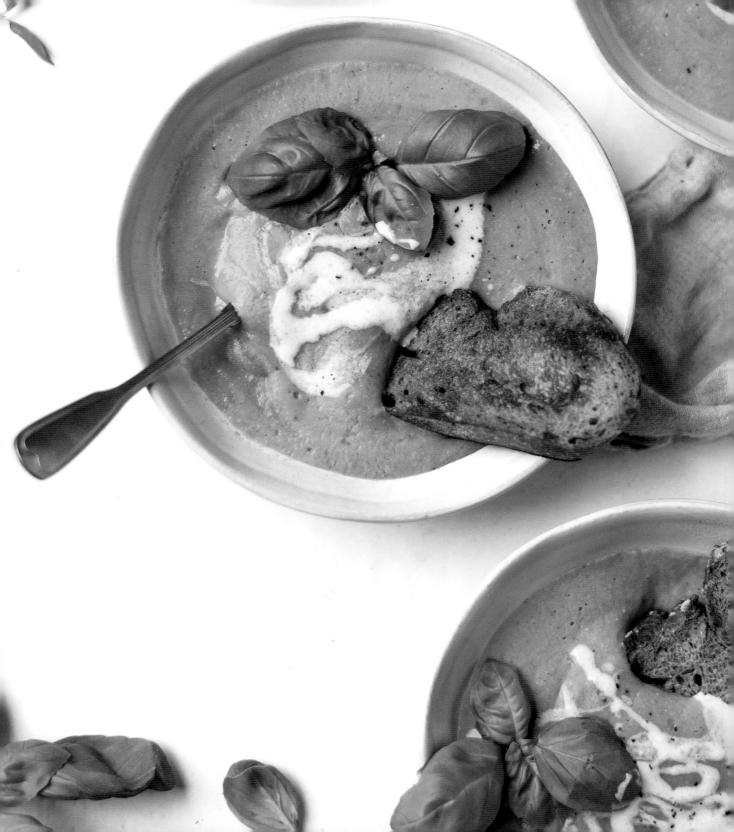

CREAMY TOMATO SOUP
PLANT PROTEIN

SERVES 2 • This is a classic recipe with tomatoes and red bell pepper. Tomato soup is an excellent source of antioxidants, flavonoids, and vitamins C and E, among many others. Tomatoes are rich in carotenoids—namely lycopene—providing about 80 percent of lycopene's recommended daily intake. The pigment that gives tomatoes their characteristic bright red color, lycopene is the most powerful antioxidant among carotenoids. The cashews make the soup creamy, and the pea protein powder lends the soup a nice structure. Serve with a slice of gluten-free bread for extra comfort on a cold or rainy day. Top with a swirl of vegan yogurt, basil leaves, and nutritional yeast.

1 white onion, diced

2 garlic cloves, minced

4 tomatoes, diced

1 red bell pepper, seeded and diced

⅓ cup tomato paste

4 tablespoons vegetable broth or hot water

2 teaspoons dried Italian herbs

2 tablespoons pea protein powder

Sea salt and pepper to taste

½ cup cashews

IN a large saucepan, heat ¼ cup water over high heat. Add the onion and garlic, and let them sizzle for 2 minutes.

ADD the tomatoes and bell pepper. After 5 minutes, add the tomato paste, broth, Italian herbs, pea protein powder, and salt and pepper to taste and stir to combine, cooking for another 10 minutes.

LADLE everything from the pan into a high-speed blender, add the cashews, and process for 1 or 2 minutes or until smooth. Add more cashews for extra creaminess.

ADD vegan yogurt, fresh basil, and/or nutritional yeast to garnish, if desired. Serve warm.

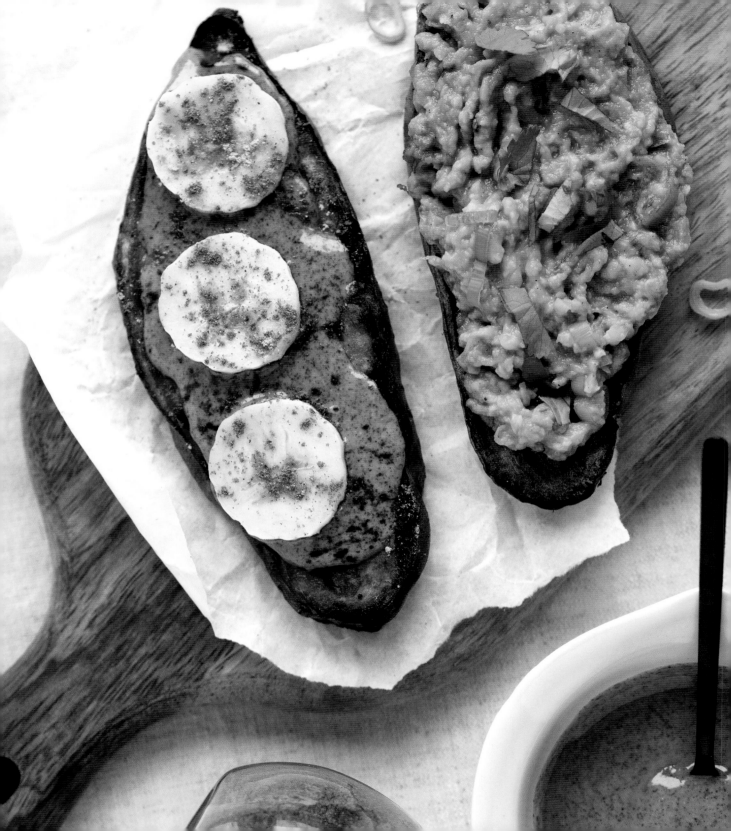

SWEET POTATO TOASTS
IMMUNITY & ENERGY

SERVES 2 • Here's our twist on avocado toast with baked sweet potatoes in place of bread. These are two of our favorite ways to top sweet potatoes, but switch it up with your favorite toast toppings. For a quick weekday lunch, bake several slices of sweet potato ahead of time, then store them in an airtight container in the refrigerator until you're ready to make your sweet potato toast. Simply pop a slice or two of your pre-baked sweet potato slabs into a toaster (yes, upright in a toaster!) or a toaster oven and "cook" until they're warm and crisp on the edges.

1 large sweet potato

SWEET AND NUTTY TOPPINGS | IMMUNITY

2 tablespoons almond butter

½ banana, sliced

1 teaspoon cinnamon powder

½ teaspoon ginger powder

CREAMY AND SAVORY TOPPINGS | ENERGY

½ avocado, sliced

¼ teaspoon matcha powder

1 scallion, sliced

Sea salt and pepper to taste

Cilantro, chopped, optional

PREHEAT the oven to 400°F.

SLICE the sweet potato lengthwise into even slices (approximately ¼- to ½-inch thick) using a knife.

SPREAD the slices on parchment paper and roast in the oven for 15 or 20 minutes until soft on the inside and toasty on the outside.

FOR Sweet and Nutty toast, spread the almond butter on the sweet potato slices, then top with banana slices and sprinkle with cinnamon and ginger.

FOR Creamy and Savory toast, spread the avocado on the sweet potatoes and mash them a bit with a fork. Sprinkle with matcha, scallion, and salt and pepper. Garnish with cilantro, if using.

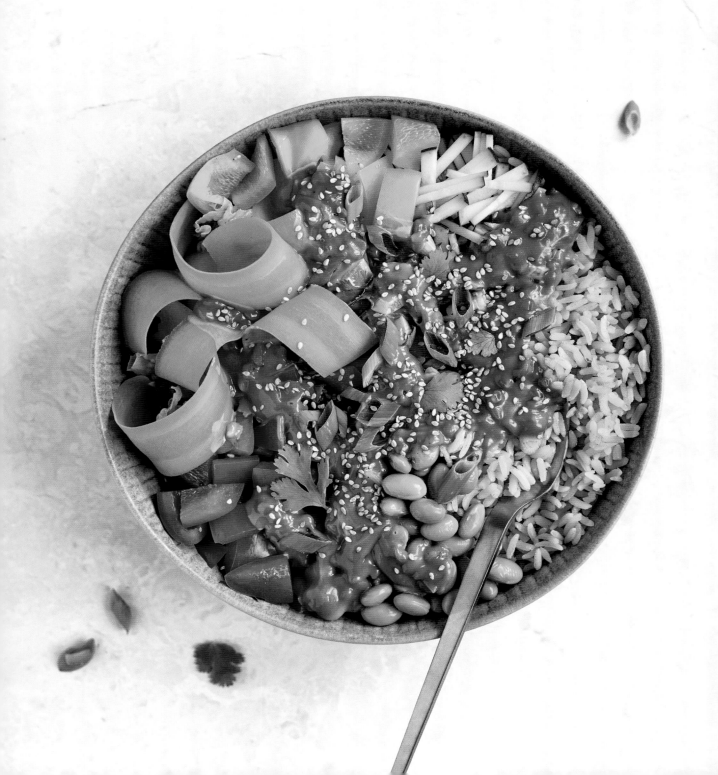

THAI-INSPIRED PEANUT SALAD

STRESS REDUCTION & IMMUNITY

SERVES 1 • This protein-packed salad is topped with a creamy Thai-inspired dressing made with peanut butter, garlic, and tamari. We like to buy frozen edamame beans, as they're easy to steam for a minute, and perfect in salads or even simply as a high-protein snack. Edamame beans are whole, immature soybeans. A cup of cooked edamame provides around 18.5 grams of protein. Unlike most plant proteins, they provide all the essential amino acids your body needs. Edamame is rich in several vitamins and minerals, especially vitamin K and folate.

1 cup frozen edamame beans

½ cup cooked brown rice

1 carrot, sliced

¼ zucchini, diced

½ red and/or yellow bell pepper, seeded and diced

½ head romaine lettuce, chopped

Cilantro, chopped

2 scallions, sliced

PEANUT DRESSING

2 tablespoons peanut butter

1 garlic clove, minced

1 teaspoon maple syrup

1 tablespoon tamari sauce

½ teaspoon reishi powder, optional

Sea salt and pepper to taste

IN a pan with a thin layer of water over medium heat, steam frozen edamame beans until thawed and warm.

COMBINE edamame with the rice and veggies.

TO make the dressing, combine all the ingredients in a small glass and stir together with a fork until smooth.

DRIZZLE the dressing on top of salad.

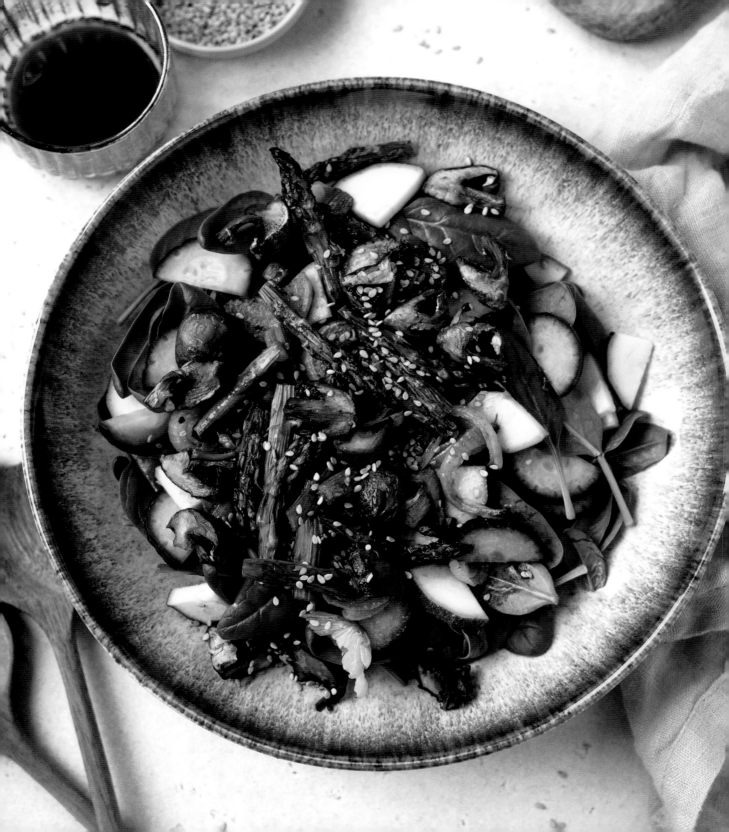

MUSHROOM SALAD
IMMUNITY & STRESS REDUCTION

SERVES 1 • The combination of roasted and raw veggies makes this salad delicious. Plus, with minimal ingredients, it's easy to make. Did you know that green asparagus can be eaten cooked or raw? Asparagus is high in folate and vitamins A, C, and K and is a good source of fiber, antioxidants, including vitamin E, and flavonoids and polyphenols. The dressing draws inspiration from Asian seasonings like tamari, ginger, and sesame oil and is salty and fresh at the same time. Powerful mushroom superfoods give you an extra health boost!

2 cups brown button mushrooms, sliced

5 green asparagus spears, sliced

1 onion, diced

DRESSING

2 tablespoons sesame oil

2 tablespoons tamari sauce

1 tablespoon maple syrup

Juice of ½ lemon

½ teaspoon ginger powder

2 cups fresh spinach

¼ green zucchini, diced

¼ cucumber, diced

½ teaspoon reishi powder, optional

½ teaspoon chaga powder, optional

½ teaspoon onion powder

Sea salt and pepper to taste

PREHEAT the oven to 400°F. Line a baking sheet with parchment paper and place the mushrooms, asparagus, and onion in a single layer on the sheet. Bake for 10 to 15 minutes.

ADD the spinach, zucchini, and cucumber to a large bowl, and top with the baked veggies.

TO make the dressing, stir all ingredients together with a fork in a glass jar. Drizzle on top of the salad and enjoy.

GERMAN POTATO SALAD
PLANT PROTEIN

SERVES 1 • This is Michael's favorite lunch. It was inspired by a salad his Grannie used to make for him. It's still creamy, filling, and delicious, but now plant-based and packed with nutrition. We use tofu instead of egg. You could also use mashed chickpeas. Did you know that adding sauerkraut to your lunch helps your probiotic intake? Even just one tablespoon of sauerkraut a day can help with your gut health! Making the first bite of your meal a bite of sauerkraut helps you digest your lunch better. You can make your own sauerkraut or use a store-bought one— just look for one without any unhealthy additives or preservatives, and buy organic if you can.

3 medium yellow potatoes, scrubbed and cubed

6 ounces firm tofu, drained and pressed

1 medium yellow onion, diced

1 cup alfalfa sprouts, optional

4 tablespoons sauerkraut, optional

SAUCE

5 tablespoons white vinegar

3 tablespoons tahini

1 teaspoon garlic powder

Sea salt and pepper to taste

2 tablespoons nutritional yeast, optional

BOIL the potatoes in a large pot of water over high heat for 20 to 25 minutes. Set aside to cool.

CUT the tofu into bite-size pieces. Combine the onions, tofu, and boiled potatoes in a large bowl.

IN a glass jar or bowl, mix together the white vinegar, tahini, garlic powder, salt and pepper, and nutritional yeast, if using, with 3 or 4 tablespoons of water to thin, then add to the potato bowl, mixing everything together by tossing well.

TOP with the sprouts and sauerkraut, if using, and serve.

HOW TO MAKE SOUP

Soup is the perfect way to pack a lot of veggies into your lunch. It's easy to prep ahead of time and it can even be a great snack! It's kind of a smoothie but made with all veggies. Making soup is easier than you think—here are five simple steps to help you come up with your own creations. Have fun trying different combinations—learning how to cook is all about trying things out and discovering the flavor combinations that you particularly love.

① CHOOSE YOUR VEGGIES

Choose 4 cups of veggies: broccoli, zucchini, cauliflower, tomatoes, mushrooms, asparagus, kohlrabi, green beans, leafy greens like spinach or kale, celery, carrots, cabbage, or bell pepper. If you want your soup to be creamy, include one or more of these: potato (sweet or regular), pumpkin, or squash. For extra protein and quick cooking, add canned beans or lentils. To pack a punch of extra flavor, add garlic cloves, onions, or leeks.

② CHOOSE YOUR BASE

Start with 4 cups of liquid: hot water, plant-based milk like coconut or almond milk, or vegetable broth. Optionally, make it extra creamy by adding 4 tablespoons nut butter like cashew or almond butter, ½ avocado, 1 cup cashews (if you're going to puree your soup), or 4 tablespoons coconut cream.

③ ADD SPICES AND SUPERFOODS

Yummy spices to add are black pepper, salt, chili powder, cumin, curry, Italian herbs, turmeric, ginger, onion, garlic, miso paste, tamari sauce, or nutritional yeast. Great savory superfoods for soups are reishi, chaga, moringa, spirulina, kelp, tulsi, hemp protein, pea protein, chlorella, baobab, ashwagandha, or shatavari.

④ COOK

Throw all the ingredients together in a large pot and boil for 15 to 30 minutes or until all veggies are soft (time will depend on your choice of veggies). Or use leftover roasted veggies and simply use these with your hot base, spices, and superfoods right away in the blender. No time for boiling needed.

⑤ TIME TO BLEND PUREED SOUPS

If you want a super smooth soup, throw it all in a blender and puree until smooth. If you want some chunks or texture, shorten your blend time and simply pulse several times or use an immersion blender. You can also play with the amount of liquid depending on whether you like a thicker or thinner soup.

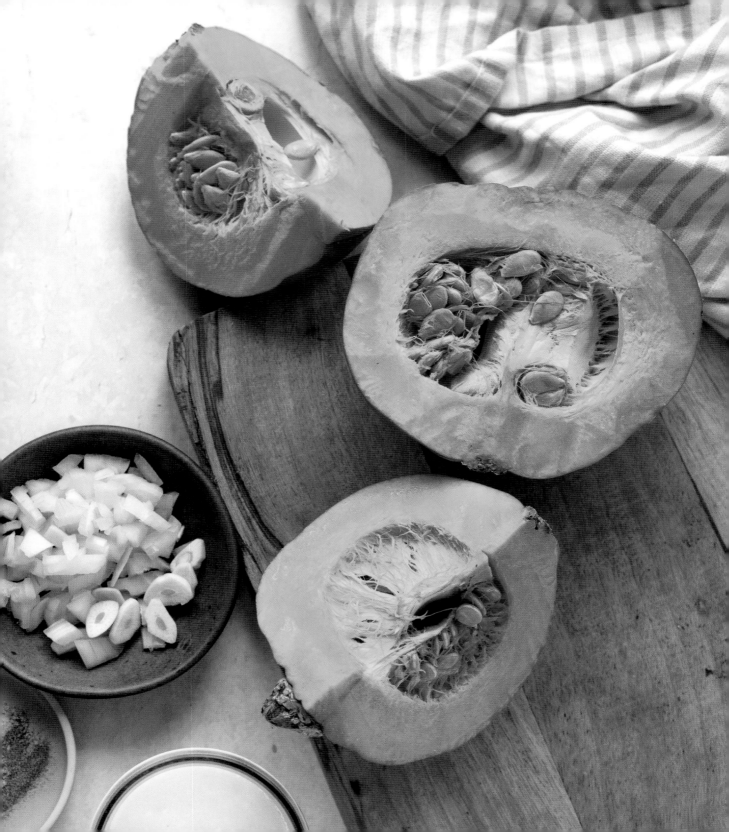

HOW TO MAKE A SALAD BOWL

Yup, we love eating lots of greens. Making salad can be easy if you know the steps. Wash and cut all your veggies, then steam, stir-fry, or oven roast whatever you don't want to eat raw, make a quick salad dressing, and toss everything together!

① CHOOSE YOUR BASE

Greens or grains? Or combine both! For a green salad, choose from spinach, mixed greens, kale, chard, or romaine lettuce. For a grain salad, choose from brown rice, quinoa, millet, buckwheat, or amaranth.

② CHOOSE YOUR VEGGIES

The sky's the limit! Cucumber, tomato, spring onion, bell peppers, broccoli, celery, beetroot, asparagus, cauliflower, carrots, and zucchini are some of our favorites to use raw. Root vegetables like pumpkin and sweet potatoes are great as well when boiled or roasted. You can make this a mix of raw and cooked, as desired.

③ CHOOSE YOUR PROTEIN

Add some healthy veggie protein: lentils, mushrooms, peas or beans, or tofu or tempeh.

④ DRESSINGS

It's all about that dressing. Dressings are perfect to hide your superfood powders in. Try adding açaí, baobab, moringa, wheatgrass, reishi, turmeric, ginger, or kelp (see superfood table, pages 22–23). Throughout the lunch chapter you'll find many of our favorite dressings. Make a large batch of your favorite to have it ready to go.

⑤ TOPPINGS

Add nuts and seeds: almonds, walnuts, pumpkin seeds, sesame seeds, sunflower seeds, or flaxseeds. And add healthy herbs like parsley, cilantro, chives, thyme, or basil as toppings.

TIPS

ADD dinner leftovers to our lunch salad the next day.

BATCH-COOK quinoa or rice to use in lunches throughout the week.

PREP your lunch the night before or in the morning and take it with you in a mason jar. We like to put the dressing at the bottom of the jar and shake everything up just before eating.

DOUBLE the recipe and you'll have lunch ready for the next two days. Just hold off on dressing the salad until you're ready to eat.

DON'T have time to make your own salad for lunch? Check and see if there's a healthy salad bar close by.

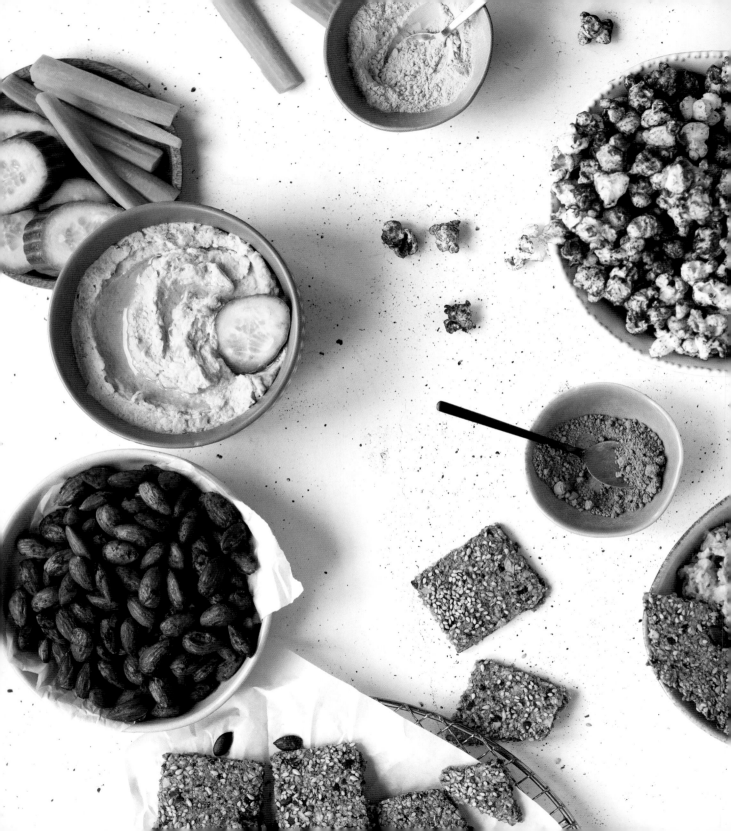

SUPPORT
HUNGER-BUSTING AFTERNOON SNACKS

Yes, more snacks! We really mean it when we say that we want to encourage you to listen to your body's cues and eat when hungry. The end of the day is a time of transition and the perfect time to nurture yourself with a satisfying snack. These delicious recipes will keep the whole family hydrated and satisfied between meals—and help you resist the effects of the day's stress on your body.

Many store-bought snacks contain a highly addictive combination of salt, sugar, and fat, and very little in the way of nutrients your body needs. Our snacks are high in nutrients and crafted with love—plus they are infinitely customizable. You can decide what powerful super plants you want to add to support your health.

We find that at this time of day we tend to crave more salty and crunchy things, like our superfood popcorn, energizing guac, and immunity-boosting hummus—and lots of water. This is often a time of day when we need plenty of hydration, so please remember to drink water. (Check out our recipes for superfood-infused waters on pages 181–184.) We've got nourishing smoothies or milkshakes, too. Most of these are easy to prep at the beginning of the week, so you have them ready when you need a pick-me-up, or can take them on the go. We also think they're perfect for sharing!

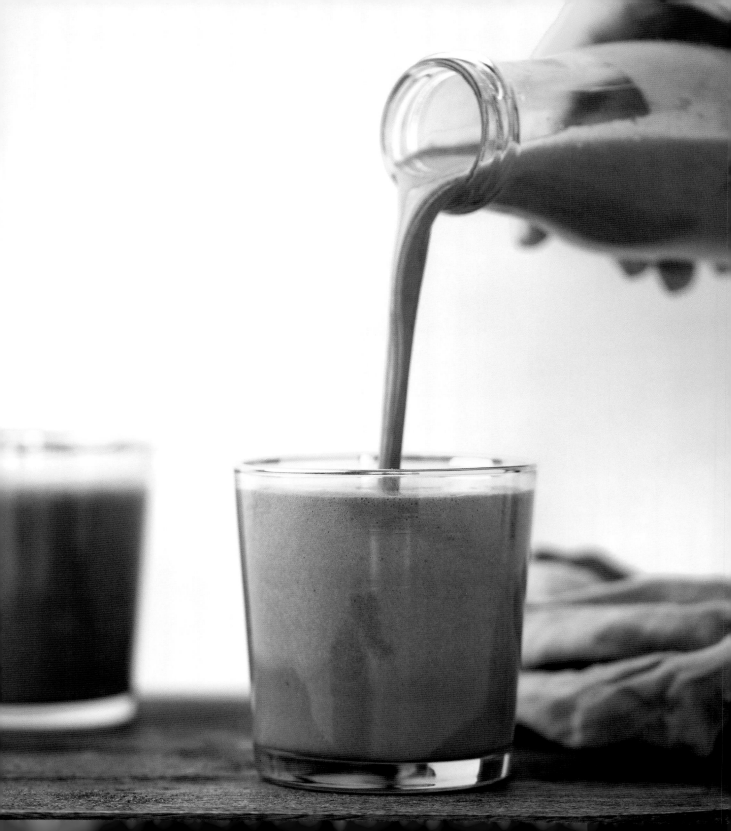

POWER CHOCO SMOOTHIE
PLANT PROTEIN & MOOD BOOSTER

SERVES 1 • This is a perfect chocolate smoothie with healthy carbs for energy, protein to keep you full longer, and healthy fats. It's the perfect afternoon snack if you are hungry and want something sweet.

2 teaspoons cacao powder

2 tablespoons pea protein powder, optional

½ teaspoon chaga powder, optional

1 frozen banana

1 tablespoon hazelnut butter

1 cup almond milk

A pinch of sea salt

BLEND all ingredients in a high-speed blender until smooth and creamy. Drink right away.

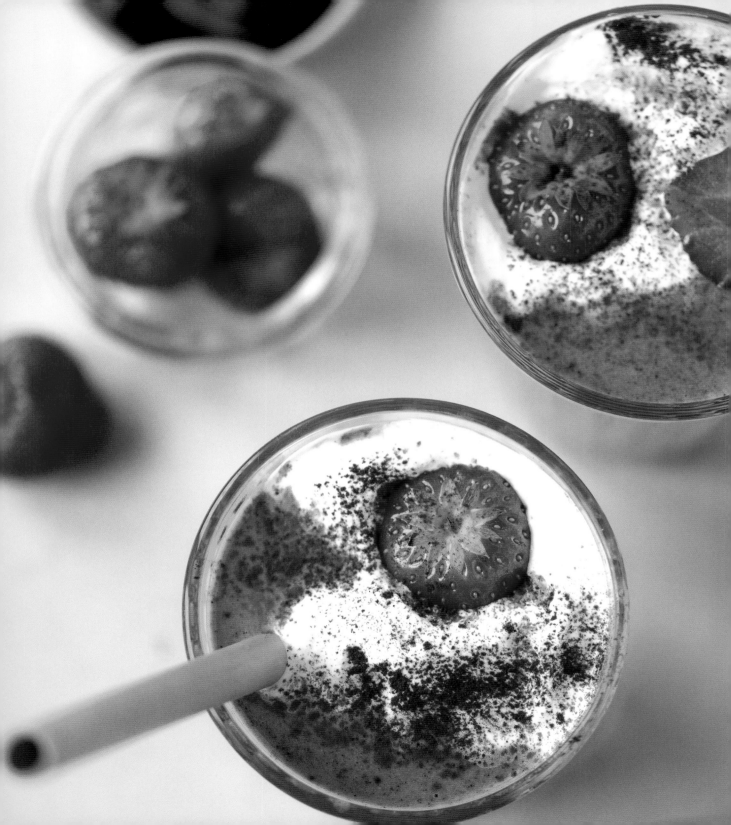

BERRYLICIOUS MILKSHAKE

HEALTHY SKIN

SERVES 1 • Who doesn't love a berry milkshake? This one won't give you the usual sugar crash a regular milkshake gives you. Instead you'll feel energized and satisfied—and it supports your skin from the inside out with powerful antioxidant-rich berries. Tocos is an incredible superfood and creamy addition to any recipe. Derived from the bran of organically grown brown rice, tocos is known as a super-rich source of fat-soluble vitamin E. Garnish with coconut cream and a little bit of cacao to make it extra special.

½ cup canned coconut milk

1 teaspoon açaí powder

1 teaspoon maqui powder, optional

2 teaspoons tocos powder, optional

1 cup frozen strawberries

3 pitted dates

½ cup ice cubes

1 teaspoon vanilla extract, optional

Dollop of coconut cream, optional

1 teaspoon cacao powder, optional

STORE a can of coconut milk in the fridge overnight and scoop only the cream from the top, if using.

BLEND all ingredients in a high-speed blender with ½ cup water until smooth and creamy. Top with coconut cream and cacao powder, if using. Drink right away.

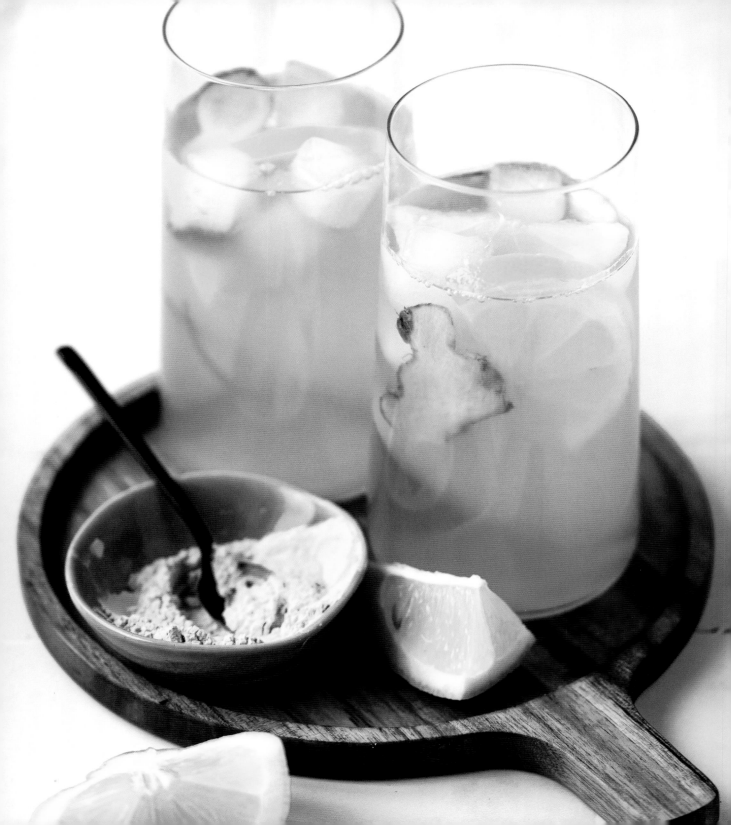

BAOBAB LEMONADE
IMMUNITY

SERVES 1 • The baobab tree is a strange-looking tree that grows in low-lying areas on the African mainland, Madagascar, and Australia. It can grow to enormous sizes, and carbon dating indicates that it may live to be 3,000 years old. Baobab fruit is high in vitamin C, a powerful antioxidant, as well as fiber to support digestive health and balance blood sugar levels. Local residents use it for energy as well. We love it in the afternoon because it's a real thirst killer—perfect for that time of day when you're running from one thing to another. Garnish with mint leaves and ice cubes.

2 teaspoons baobab powder

1½ cups coconut water

½ cup ice cubes

½ inch fresh ginger root, thinly sliced

½ lemon, sliced

SIMPLY stir everything together and enjoy this refreshing and hydrating drink!

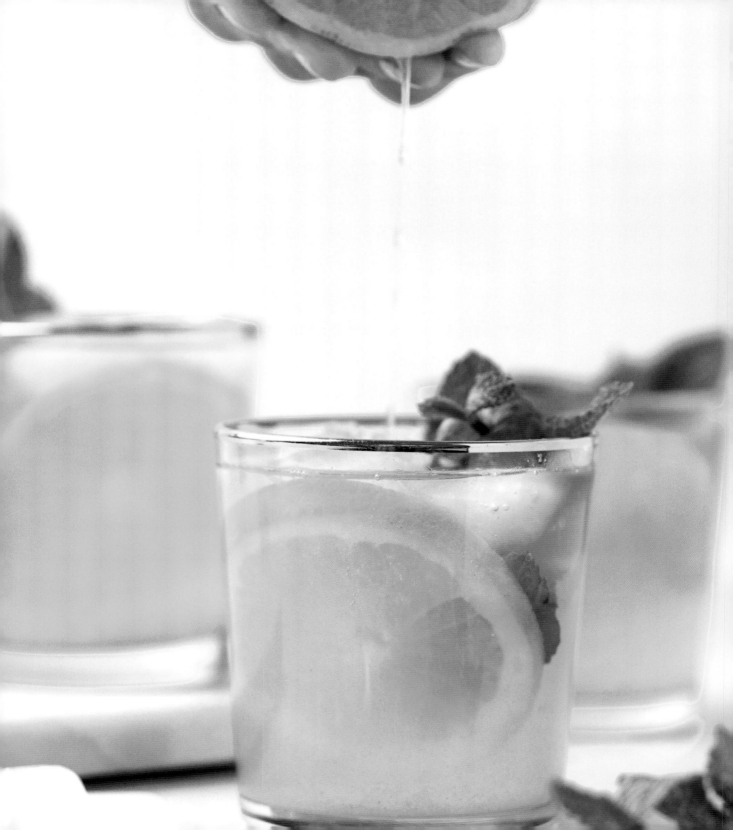

SPARKLING TURMERIC REFRESHER
ANTI-INFLAMMATORY

SERVES 1 • Sometimes we get tired of drinking water; instead of buying a soda we make our own superfood-infused bubbly drink. Curcumin is a bioactive substance that can fight inflammation. To make the curcumin in turmeric even more absorbable, it is best consumed with a little bit of pepper, which you can always sprinkle on top of your drink. The piperine in black pepper enhances the absorption of curcumin by 2,000 percent!

1½ cups of sparkling water

1 teaspoon turmeric powder

1 teaspoon maple syrup, optional

½ orange

½ cup ice cubes

STIR the turmeric into the sparkling water, and add the maple syrup, if using.

SLICE the orange into 4 equal parts. Squeeze the juice into the water and throw the squeezed rinds in the drink.

ADD the ice cubes. Stir and enjoy!

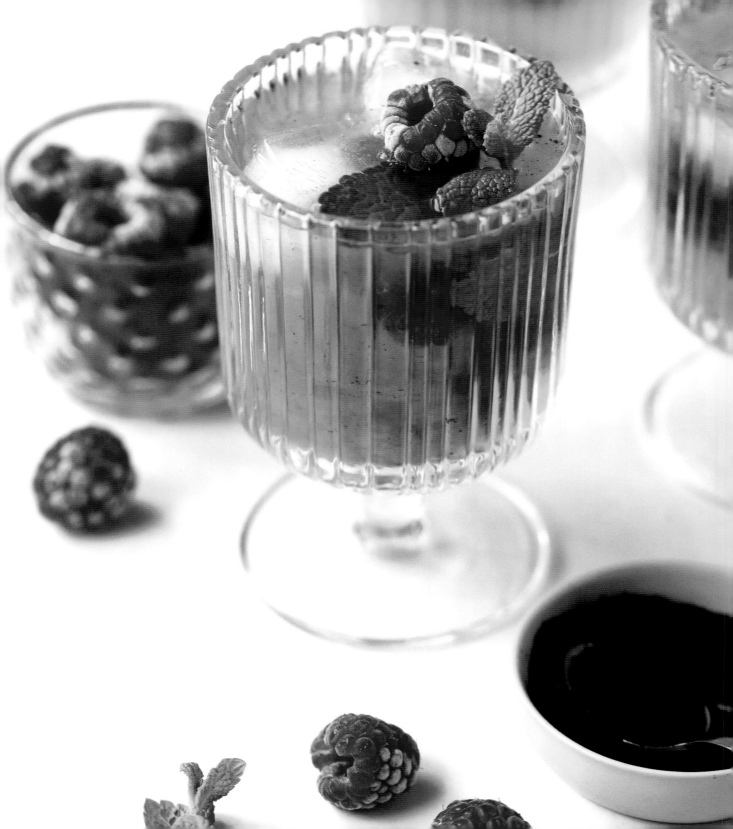

ENERGIZING BERRY WATER
ENERGY & HEALTHY SKIN

SERVES 1 • This refreshing and sweet drink is another great example of how to make your water taste good so that you stay well hydrated. Drinking enough water each day is crucial to regulating body temperature, keeping joints lubricated, preventing infections, delivering nutrients to cells, and keeping your organs functioning properly, among other functions. Being well-hydrated also improves sleep quality, cognition, and mood. But why not make your water even better with yummy infusions and superfoods?

½ teaspoon açaí powder

½ teaspoon guarana powder, optional

½ cup frozen raspberries

½ cup ice cubes

1 stalk fresh mint leaves, optional

STIR the açaí and guarana powder, if using, together in 1½ cups of water.

ADD the frozen raspberries, ice cubes, and mint leaves, if using. Stir once more before drinking.

DETOX WATER
DETOX & IMMUNITY

SERVES 1 • This is an easy way to add more greens to your day. Chlorella is single-celled, green freshwater algae that is 60 percent protein. It contains all the amino acids and is also a good source of vitamin C, iron, B vitamins, antioxidants, and omega-3. It supports detoxification, the immune system, and overall health. Be aware of where your chlorella is sourced—if it tastes fishy, it's not a high-quality source.

1 teaspoon chlorella powder
½ lemon

½ cup ice cubes
5 sliced cucumber pieces, optional

STIR chlorella into 1½ cups of water and stir.

SQUEEZE in the juice of the lemon and add the remaining rind to the water. Stir once more.

ADD ice cubes and cucumber slices, if using, and enjoy.

KIDNEY BEAN HUMMUS
HEALTHY SKIN & PLANT PROTEIN

SERVES 3 • Kristel discovered this recipe by accident one day while playing around with superfood berries and kidney beans. Kidney beans are among the best sources of plant-based protein. They're also rich in healthy fibers, which moderate blood sugar levels and promote colon and digestive health. The berries are high in antioxidants. Together they're a happy combination! Eat with crackers or fresh-cut veggies.

1 can (15 ounces) kidney beans, about 1½ cups, drained and rinsed

4 tablespoons tahini

1 teaspoon açaí powder, optional

1 teaspoon maqui powder, optional

1 teaspoon chili powder

1 teaspoon cumin powder

½ teaspoon garlic powder

Sea salt and pepper to taste

THROW all the ingredients in the high-speed blender or food processor with ½ cup of water and blend until smooth. Add more water if needed to make it more spreadable.

SERVE immediately or store in an airtight container for up to one week.

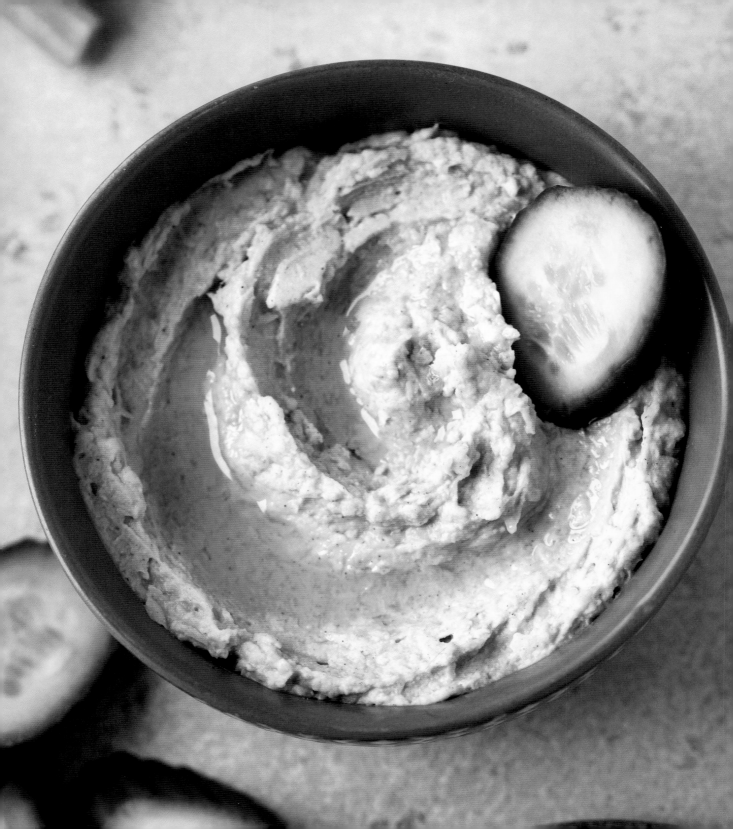

GREAT NORTHERN BEAN HUMMUS
IMMUNITY & PLANT PROTEIN

SERVES 3 • This is a delicious hummus that goes with any lunch or dinner or makes the perfect snack to dip fresh veggies or crackers in. It's a great base for adding superfoods to your diet. We like to use baobab for extra vitamin C and a brightness similar to lemon juice, but you can also spice it up with turmeric, ginger powder, reishi, or chili powder. It's a blank canvas.

1 can (15 ounces) great northern or navy beans, about 1½ cups, drained and rinsed

4 tablespoons tahini

2 teaspoons baobab powder, optional

Juice of ½ lemon

½ teaspoon garlic powder

Sea salt and pepper, to taste

THROW all the ingredients into a high-speed blender or food processor with ½ cup of water and blend until smooth. Add more water if needed to make it more spreadable.

STORE in a closed container in the fridge for up to 3 days.

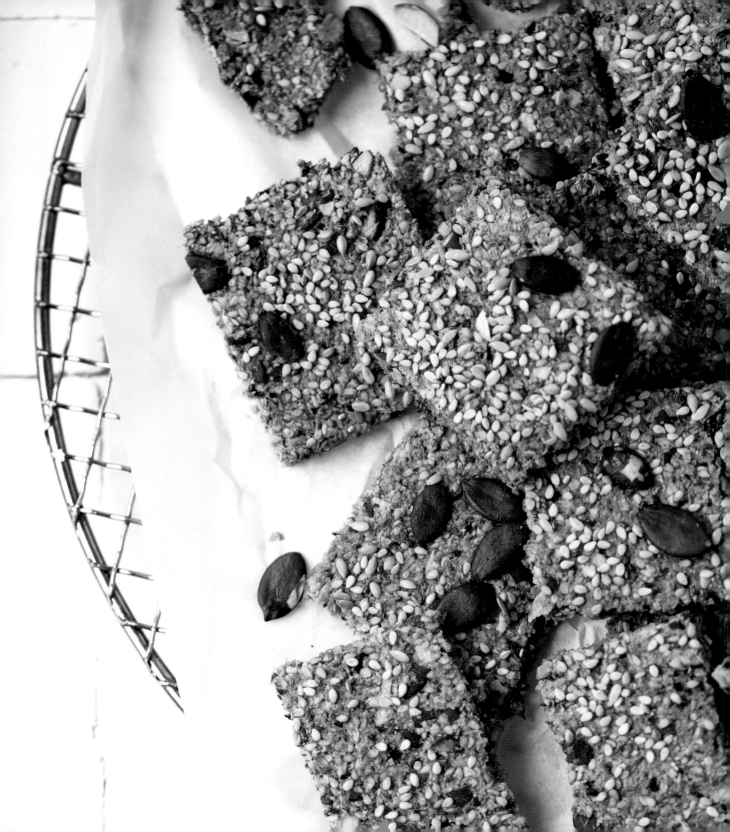

SUPERFOOD CRACKERS
HEALTHY FATS & DETOX

SERVES 4 • These easy crackers are great by themselves or dip them into hummus or your favorite dip. Seeds like flax and chia are loaded with healthy fats and fiber. They also contain many important vitamins, minerals, and antioxidants. I added moringa for extra greens, but you can switch them up by adding mushrooms, other greens, or turmeric.

½ cup pumpkin seeds

1 cup ground flaxseeds

⅓ cup sesame seeds

¼ cup chia seeds

1 teaspoon salt

1 teaspoon garlic powder

1 teaspoon onion powder

1 teaspoon italian seasoning

2 teaspoon moringa powder, optional

Sea salt and pepper to taste

PREHEAT the oven to 200°F. Line a baking sheet with parchment paper.

COMBINE all ingredients in a high-speed blender or food processor with ½ cup water and pulse until well blended.

SPOON the mixture onto your lined baking sheet and spread out evenly, as thinly as possible.

BAKE for about 30 minutes until dry and crispy.

LET cool completely, then break them up. Store for 1 week in a sealed container.

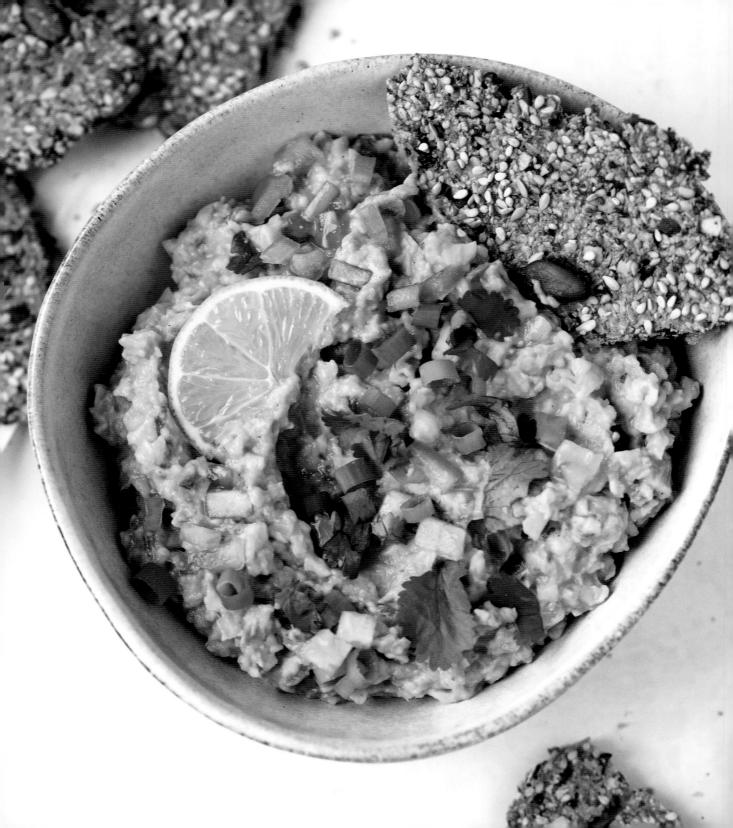

ENERGY GUAC
ENERGY & HEALTHY FATS

SERVES 3 • This recipe is a match(a) made in heaven: energy-boosting matcha powder with nutrient-rich avocados. The fiber and healthy fats will help you feel full between meals. Other superfoods like wheatgrass or moringa work well here, too!

2 avocados, pitted

½ tomato, diced

½ teaspoon matcha powder, optional

2 green onions, chopped

Cilantro, finely chopped, optional

Juice of ½ lime

½ teaspoon chili powder

Sea salt and pepper to taste

SCOOP out the avocado and place in a bowl.

ADD the tomato, matcha, green onions, and cilantro, if using.

SQUEEZE lime juice over the veggies, and add chili powder and salt and pepper.

STIR everything together with a fork, mashing the avocado as you go. Serve immediately with fresh veggies like carrots and celery or flaxseed crackers. Store in the fridge in an airtight container, adding extra lime juice to prevent browning.

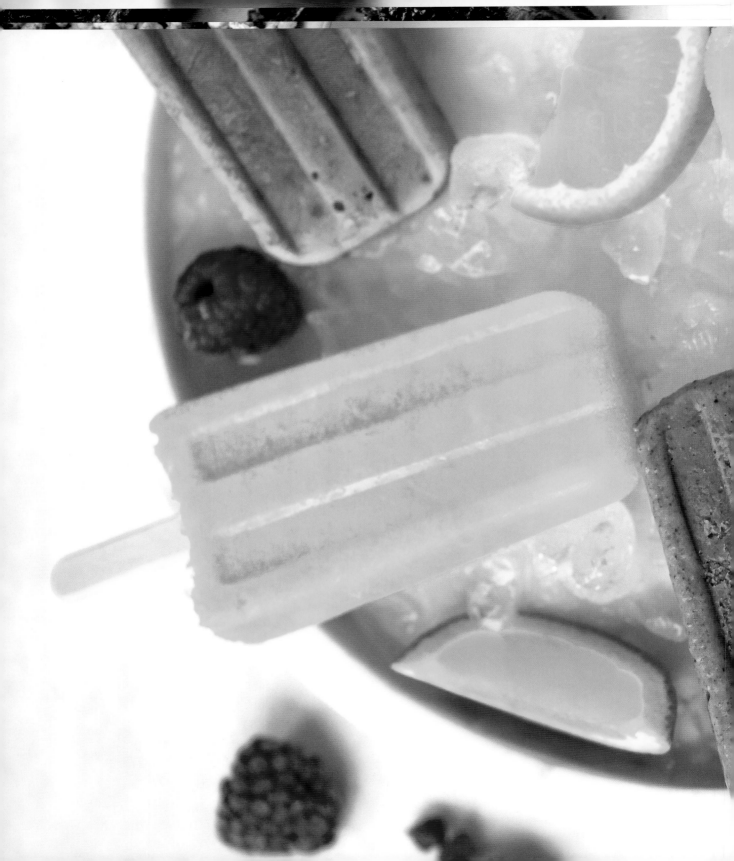

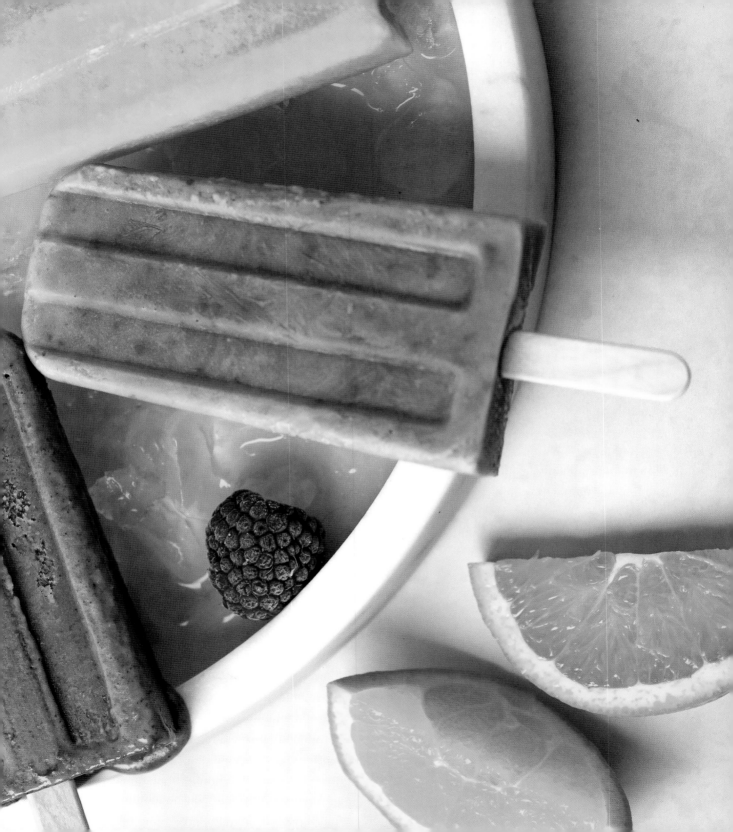

SUPER POPS

IMMUNITY & ANTI-INFLAMMATORY & HORMONE HEALTH & STRESS REDUCTION

SERVES 2 • Superfood ice pops are really just frozen smoothies to have on hand for whenever you crave a treat! The green pop is refreshing, the yellow pop is a little spicy with ginger and turmeric, the pink pop is creamy, and the chocolate pop is indulgent and helps you calm down.

GREEN LEMON POP | IMMUNITY

1 teaspoon wheatgrass powder

1 teaspoon baobab powder, optional

Juice of 1 lemon

1 tablespoon maple syrup

1 cup water

YELLOW POP | ANTI-INFLAMMATORY

½ teaspoon turmeric powder

½ teaspoon ginger powder

1 orange

1 tablespoon maple syrup

1 cup water

PINK POP | HORMONE HEALTH

1 cup frozen raspberries

½ can canned coconut milk

1 teaspoon maca powder

½ teaspoon shatavari powder, optional

1 tablespoon maple syrup

CHOCOLATE POP | STRESS REDUCTION

1 banana

1 tablespoon almond butter

2 teaspoons cacao powder

½ teaspoon ashwagandha powder, optional

1 cup almond milk

1 tablespoon maple syrup

BLEND all the ingredients in a high-speed blender until smooth and pour into ice pop molds.

FREEZE overnight. When ready to eat, run the mold under hot water to loosen the pop.

ROASTED CHICKPEAS
ANTI-INFLAMMATORY & PLANT PROTEIN

SERVES 3 • Chickpeas, also known as garbanzo beans, have been grown and eaten in Middle Eastern countries for thousands of years. The protein and fiber in chickpeas may help keep your appetite under control. Wonder if you need to eat more fiber? On average, American adults eat 10 to 15 grams of total fiber per day, while the USDA's recommended daily amount for adults up to age 50 is 25 grams for women and 38 grams for men.[1]

½ teaspoon turmeric powder

½ teaspoon ginger powder

½ teaspoon garlic powder

1 teaspoon curry powder

½ teaspoon ashwagandha powder, optional

1 can (15 ounces) chickpeas, about 1½ cups, drained and rinsed

1 tablespoon melted coconut oil

PREHEAT the oven to 400°F. Line a baking sheet with parchment paper.

MIX together all the powders.

IN a bowl combine the chickpeas, coconut oil, and powder mix. Mix well.

SPREAD the chickpeas in a single layer on your lined baking sheet and bake for about 15 minutes until crispy.

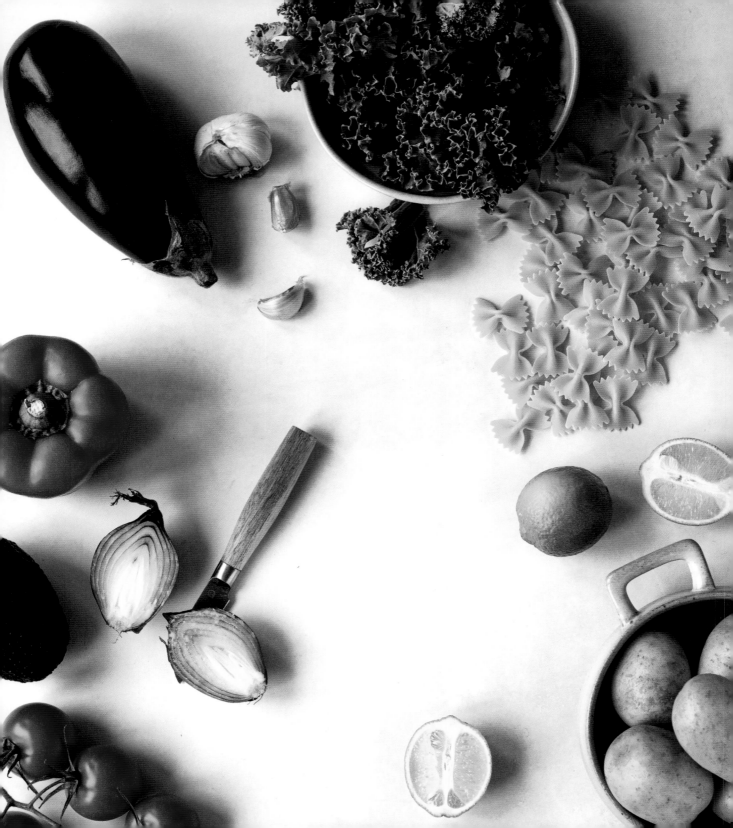

NOURISH
MAKING DINNER A HEALING RITUAL

Dinnertime is our favorite time of day because it's one of the few times we have to really connect. Cooking is a ritual we share, and our dinners have become some of the most important times we spend together. It wasn't always that way, though. At one point while building our business, we both experienced severe burnout that almost destroyed everything we had worked so hard to build. Committing to making dinnertime a ritual of unplugging and connecting with each other changed all of that.

In modern life, cooking and even eating are often viewed as chores rather than as sources of pleasure. Shopping for fresh ingredients and spending time to prepare a delicious meal can be an enjoyable experience if you change your mindset and if you have recipes for satisfying superpowered meals. Think of dinner as a time to nourish and connect with family, friends, or even yourself. Cooking can feel very meditative. In fact, your digestion starts working when you are cooking a meal—it's your body getting ready to receive nutrients from your food. If possible, take a moment during dinner prep: Be present. Put away your phone and other screens. Take time to sit down when your meal is ready and savor it.

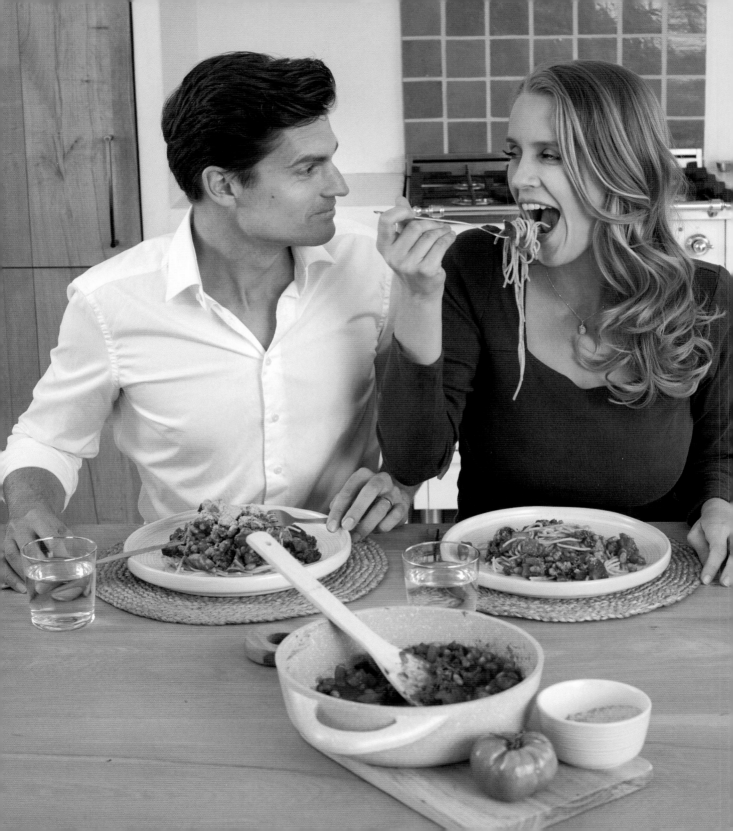

Our dinner recipes focus on simplicity and comfort. This is a collection of our favorite warm, nourishing meals you can make in just twenty to thirty minutes, making them perfect for busy workdays when you don't have hours to spare. These meals are a perfect balance of veggies; plant protein like beans, tofu, or tempeh; healthy carbs like rice, potatoes, or gluten-free pasta; superfoods; and delicious spices that bring the meal together. You'll find a variety of Italian-, East Asian-, Indian-, and Mexican-inspired flavors. (Need a refresher on staples to keep on hand for easy weeknight cooking? See pages 38–39, 41–42, and 44–45.) Experiment with these dinners, and once you find your favorites, you can add them into your regular rotation, so you always have a nourishing and filling way to end the day.

You'll notice that we mostly use water instead of oil to stir-fry. Use the water like you use oil, adding a little bit when it evaporates. We do this because oils are often processed and we don't need them much in our diet. We prefer to get healthy fats from whole food sources like avocados, nuts, or seeds. The trick is using a good ceramic-coated nonstick pan.

Kristel learned to cook from her mom, often joining her in the kitchen. Those times of connection and togetherness are some of her favorite childhood memories, and what still inspires Kristel's passion for creating new recipes today. We hope you feel that love, passion, and sense of family in our comforting dinner recipes.

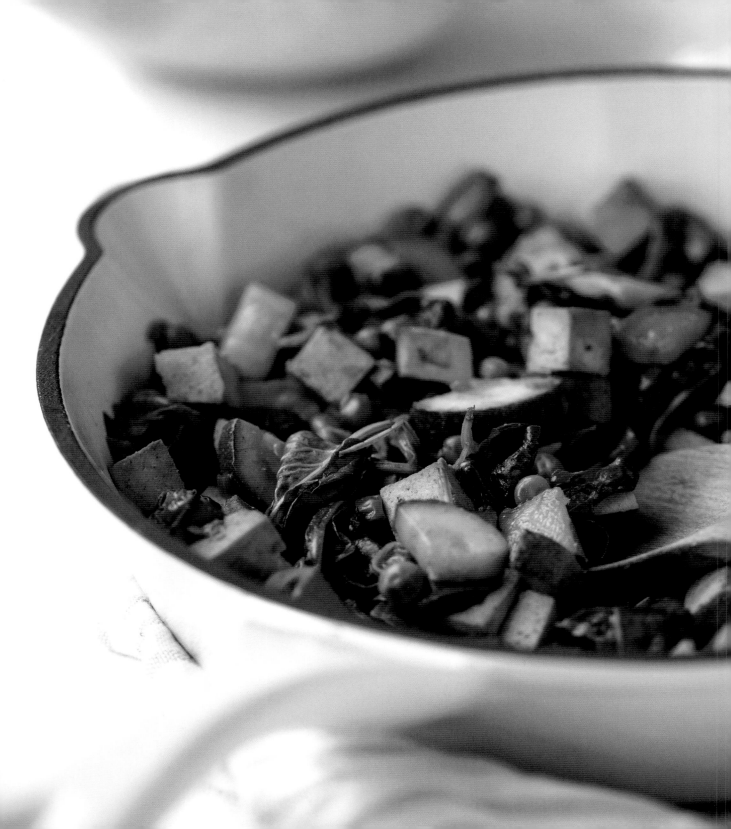

EASY GREEN STIR-FRY
IMMUNITY & DETOX

SERVES 2 • This Chinese-inspired stir-fry can be prepared with a variety of different vegetables, so if you have different veggies in the fridge, don't be afraid to mix it up. You could add brown rice or potatoes if you want something even more filling. Adding 1 or 2 teaspoons of a green superfood like spirulina right after you turn off the heat is also a great option! The tahini is our secret ingredient to make this stir-fry super indulgent. It makes it more creamy and gives it a subtle nutty taste that we love.

1 white onion, diced

1 inch fresh ginger root, thinly sliced

1 zucchini, halved and sliced into half-moons

6 ounces firm tofu, drained, pressed, and cubed

1 cup frozen peas

1 teaspoon turmeric powder

2 tablespoons tamari

½ teaspoon garlic powder

Pepper to taste

2 tablespoons tahini

3 cups fresh spinach, chopped

HEAT ½ cup water in a large ceramic-coated frying pan over high heat. Add the onion and ginger and sauté for 3 minutes.

ADD the zucchini to the pan. Stir to combine and continue stir-frying for another 5 minutes. Add more water if needed.

ADD tofu and frozen peas to the pan. Stir to combine and stir-fry for another 5 minutes.

ADD the spices: turmeric powder, tamari, garlic powder, pepper, and tahini. Add the spinach and stir-fry for another 3 minutes until tender. Serve hot.

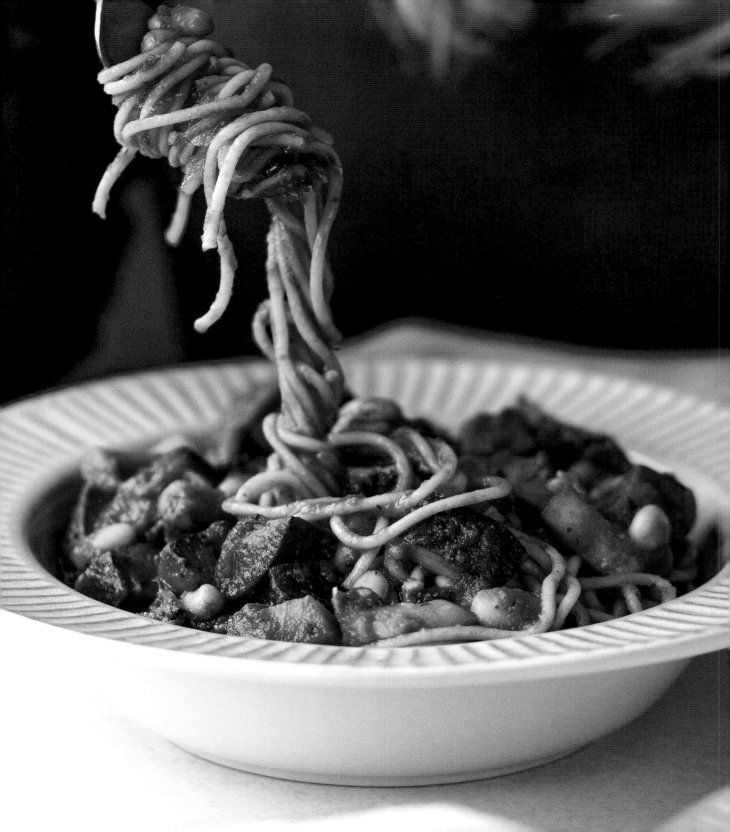

EGGPLANT PASTA
DETOX & IMMUNITY

SERVES 2 • I love making a quick pasta sauce with a bunch of veggies and pouring it over gluten-free noodles. There are so many gluten-free pasta options these days: rice, bean, lentil, quinoa, and corn pasta—experiment and find your favorite! I add a teaspoon of wheatgrass to this recipe, but you can pick any of the other green superfoods. Top with a dollop of tahini, nutritional yeast, and fresh basil leaves.

8-ounce package gluten-free pasta

1 white onion, diced

1 large eggplants, sliced into ½-inch cubes

Pinch of sea salt, plus more to taste

½ zucchini, sliced into ½-inch cubes

¾ cup tomato paste

½ teaspoon garlic powder

1 teaspoon dried oregano

Pepper to taste

1 can (15 ounces) white beans, about 1½ cups, drained and rinsed

5 kale leaves, chopped

2 teaspoons wheatgrass powder, optional

COOK the pasta according to the instructions on the package.

ADD ¼ cup of water to a large ceramic-coated frying pan over high heat. Add the onion and eggplant with a pinch of salt and cook, stirring occasionally, for 5 minutes.

ADD a cup of water and the zucchini, tomato paste, garlic powder, oregano, and pepper. Cook, stirring frequently, for about 5 minutes.

ADD the beans and the kale and cook, stirring frequently, for 2 more minutes.

TURN the heat off and stir in the wheatgrass. Pour the sauce over your cooked pasta, and serve.

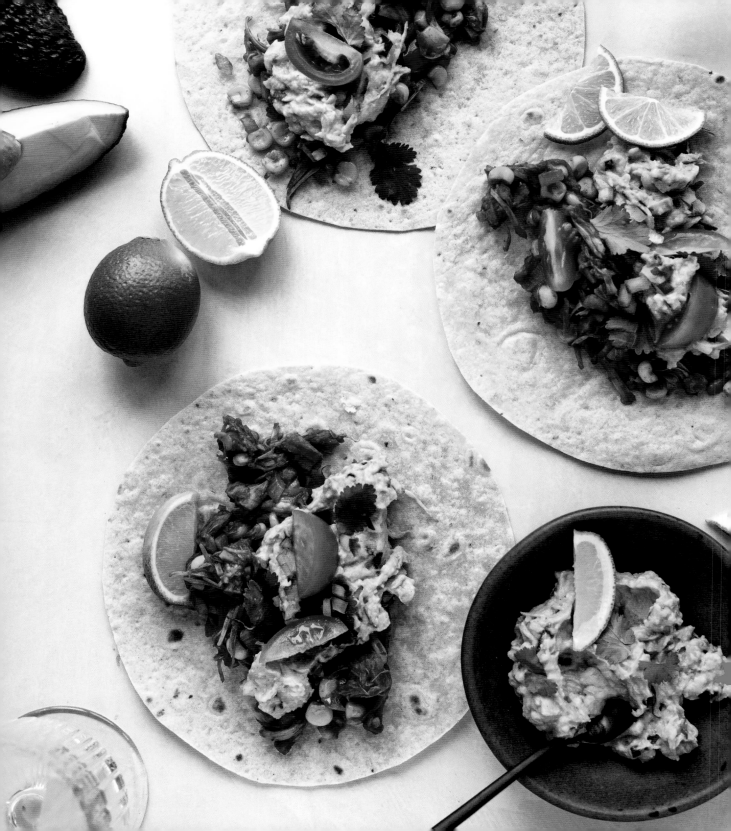

EASY TACOS

DETOX

SERVES 2 • Moringa has seven times the amount of iron as spinach! It tastes slightly sweet and bitter and is easy to hide in your dinner dishes. Jackfruit is a popular meat substitute because its texture is comparable to shredded meat. You can buy canned jackfruit in most organic supermarkets. If you can't find a clean sriracha sauce (like Yellowbird), sub chili powder instead.

TACO FILLING

½ onion, diced

1 tomato, diced

1 can (14 ounces) jackfruit, 1½ cups

⅓ cup tomato paste

1 cup frozen corn

½ teaspoon garlic powder

1 tablespoon sriracha sauce

Sea salt and pepper, to taste

6 small corn tacos

MASHED AVOCADO

1 avocado, pitted

½ onion, sliced

Juice of ½ lime

½ teaspoon moringa powder, optional

½ teaspoon chili powder

Sea salt and pepper, to taste

5 stalks fresh cilantro, chopped

HEAT ½ cup water in a large ceramic-coated frying pan over medium heat and sauté the onion for about 3 minutes.

ADD the tomato, jackfruit, tomato paste, corn, garlic, sriracha, and salt and pepper. Cook, stirring frequently, for 5 to 10 minutes until everything is heated through.

TO make the mashed avocado, scoop out the avocado flesh into a small bowl. Add all the other ingredients and mash together with a fork.

TO serve, spoon 3 tablespoons of the jackfruit mixture into a corn taco and top with the mashed avocado.

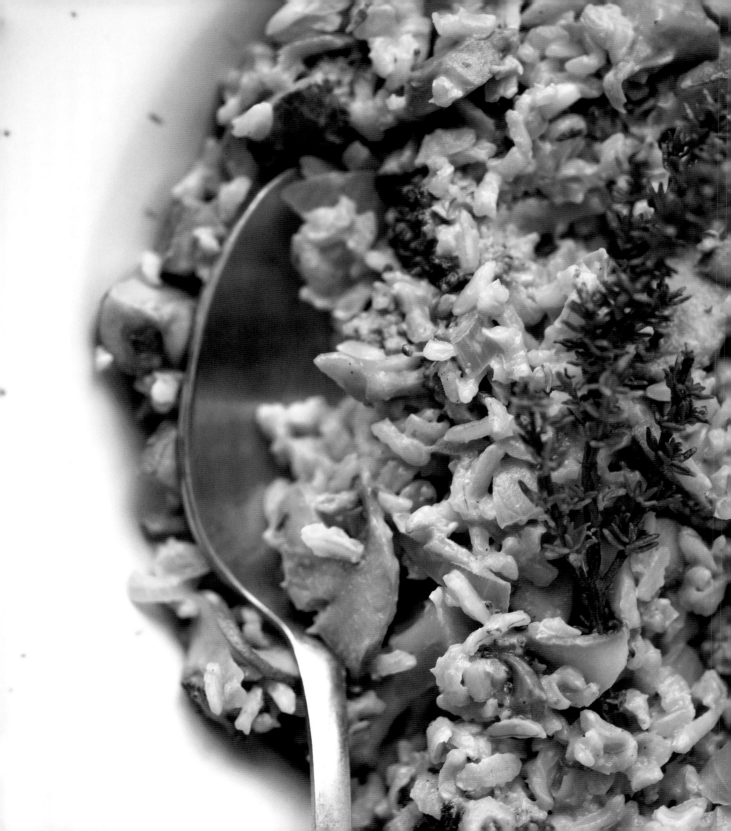

MUSHROOM RISOTTO
IMMUNITY & STRESS REDUCTION

SERVES 2 • The beauty of our take on risotto is that it's much healthier than your standard risotto—and doesn't take as long to make. It's creamy and comforting and all about the mushrooms—reishi and chaga mushroom powders combined with fresh 'shrooms of your choice. Feel free to pick your favorites—they each have a unique look and taste. The most common types found in grocery stores are shiitake, portobello, cremini, button or white mushrooms, oyster, enoki, beech, and maitake. Brush the dirt off and rinse them lightly when you're ready to use them. Mushrooms are fat-free, low-sodium, low-calorie, and cholesterol-free. They're also packed with fiber, vitamins, and minerals . . . antioxidants, B vitamins, copper, potassium, and even several cancer-fighting compounds such as a type of fiber called beta-glucan.[1]

1 onion, diced

4 cloves garlic, peeled and chopped

3 cups mushrooms of your choice

½ teaspoon reishi powder, optional

½ teaspoon chaga powder, optional

¼ teaspoon pepper

1 tablespoon tamari

½ cup canned coconut milk

½ head broccoli, chopped into bite-size florets

2 cups cooked brown rice

Thyme, optional

ADD ½ cup of water to a large ceramic-coated frying pan over high heat.

ADD the onion and garlic and sauté for 3 minutes.

ADD the mushrooms to the pan and simmer for 5 minutes.

ADD the reishi and chaga mushroom powders, if using, as well as the pepper, tamari, coconut milk, broccoli, and brown rice and stir-fry until the broccoli is cooked through, adding a little more water as needed.

GARNISH with thyme if you like and serve.

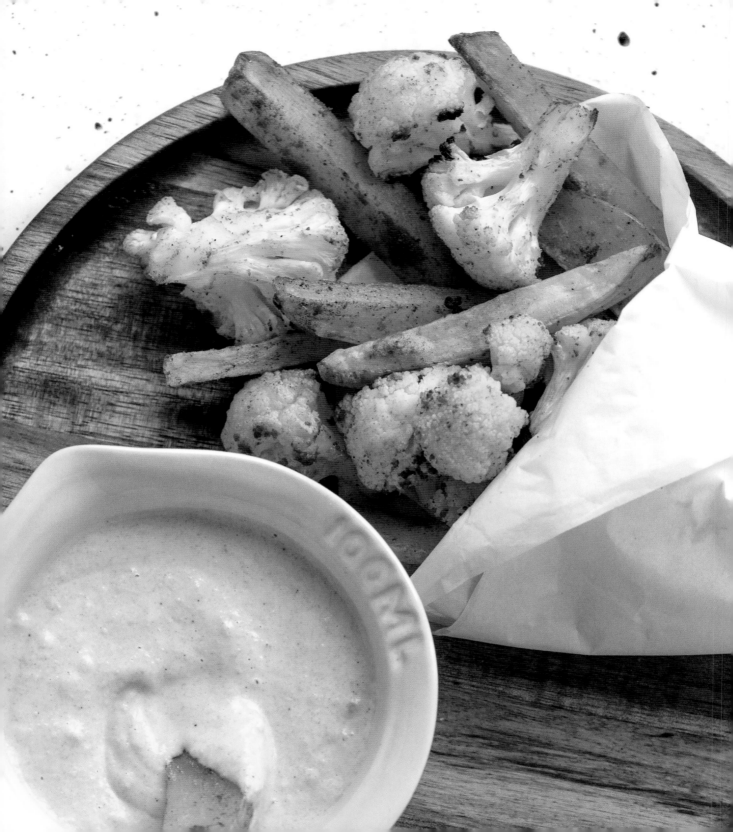

CHEESY CAULIFLOWER AND FRIES
ANTI-INFLAMMATORY & STRESS REDUCTION

SERVES 3 • This is one of our favorite dinners. It's super easy to make and, when combined with your favorite salad, it's a quick and satisfying meal. . The turmeric in the sauce is anti-inflammatory and high in curcumin, while ashwagandha helps you wind down and feel calm at the end of the day. Use the broil or roast option on your oven to make the fries crispy. You can roast them directly on the oven rack with parchment paper (instead of on a baking sheet) so the air can flow better.

1 head cauliflower, cut into bite-size chunks

17 ounces potatoes of your choice (yellow or red work well), sliced into fry shape

1 teaspoon curry powder

Sea salt and pepper

CHEESE SAUCE

6 tablespoons tahini

Juice of ½ lemon

½ teaspoon turmeric powder

2 tablespoons nutritional yeast

¼ teaspoon ashwagandha powder, optional

TAKE out an oven rack and line it with parchment paper. Preheat the oven to 400°F on the broiling or roasting function.

SPREAD the veggies on the parchment paper–covered oven rack. Sprinkle the curry powder over the cauliflower. Add some salt and pepper to taste.

ROAST for 20 to 30 minutes until golden brown and crispy.

MEANWHILE, stir the tahini, lemon juice, turmeric, nutritional yeast, and ashwagandha, if using, in a glass with a fork, for 1 or 2 minutes. Add water as needed to thin into a creamy but spreadable mixture.

DIP your fries and the cauliflower into the cheesy sauce.

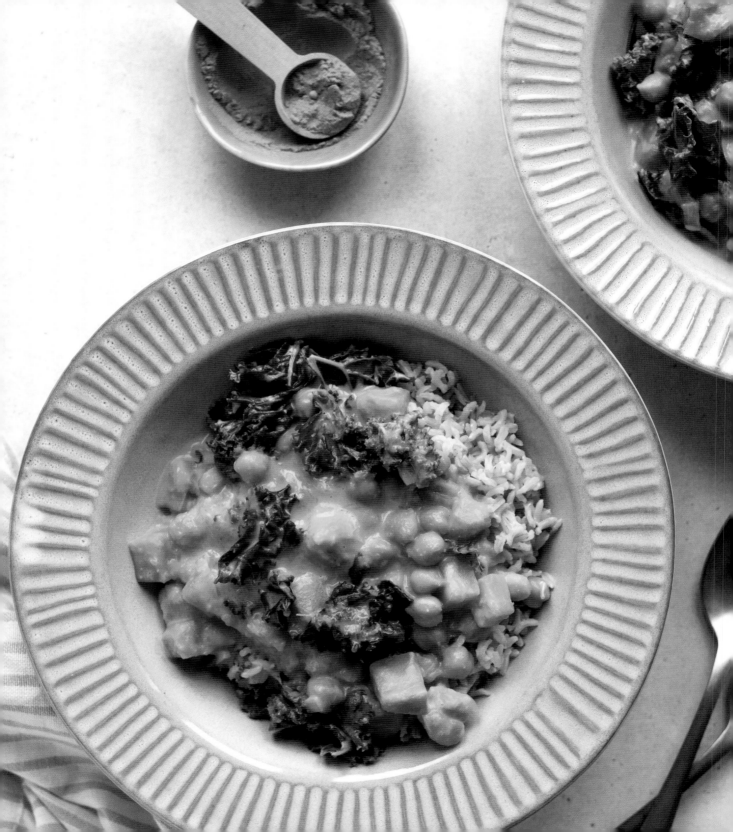

EASY PUMPKIN CURRY
ANTI-INFLAMMATORY & IMMUNITY

SERVES 3 • This warming dinner is inspired by the delicious flavors of Indian curry. Choose your favorite orange pumpkin or squash for this comforting dish. Pumpkin contains vitamin A and antioxidants such as beta-carotene and beta-cryptoxanthin. If cooked long enough, pumpkin falls apart and makes for a delicious creamy curry. You do not have to remove the skin of most pumpkins to cook them, as the majority of nutrients are found right under the skin.

3 cups cooked brown rice

1 medium-sized butternut squash or small pumpkin

1 onion, diced

2 inches fresh ginger root, chopped

1 tablespoon curry powder

1 teaspoon garlic powder

2 teaspoons turmeric powder

Sea salt and pepper, to taste

1½ cups canned coconut milk

1 can (15 ounces) chickpeas, about 1½ cups, drained and rinsed

3 cups kale, destemmed and chopped

2 teaspoons tulsi powder, optional

COOK the brown rice according to the package directions.

WASH and cut the squash or pumpkin. Remove the seeds and cut into small, 1-inch cubes. The smaller the cut, the faster it will cook.

IN a deep wok or large ceramic-coated frying pan place 1 cup of water and the onion and squash over high heat. Add ½ cup of water every 5 minutes to keep the squash about half covered with water.

ADD the ginger, curry powder, garlic powder, turmeric, and salt and pepper and continue cooking for another 15 to 20 minutes until the squash starts to soften.

ADD the coconut milk and chickpeas and continue cooking.

WHEN the pumpkin easily breaks when pierced with a fork, add the kale and tulsi. Stir with a wooden spoon, breaking the pumpkin up to create a creamier mixture. Remove from the heat after 2 minutes. Serve over rice.

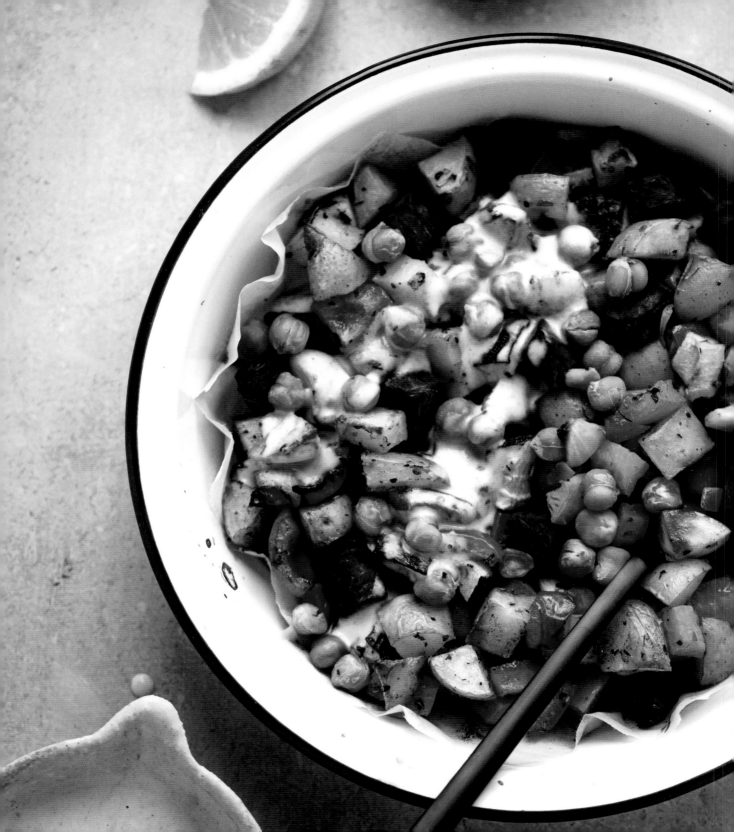

ROASTED RAINBOW VEGGIES
IMMUNITY

SERVES 3 • It's easy to forget how good simple roasted veggies can be. If you ever don't know what to cook, pick up whatever veggies you have and throw them in the oven. Many people think you need to use oil when roasting veggies, but you don't have to! I mainly roast veggies on my oven's broil option without any oil. Make extra so you have leftovers to toss on your salad for lunch the next day.

3 potatoes, cut into 1-inch cubes

2 large carrots, cut into 1-inch cubes

1 raw beet, washed and cut into 1-inch cubes

1 zucchini, cut into 1-inch cubes

1 red bell pepper, cut into 1-inch cubes

1 onion, diced

6 garlic cloves, peeled

1 can (15 ounces) chickpeas, about 1½ cups, drained and rinsed

3 teaspoons dried Italian herbs

Sea salt and pepper, to taste

SUPERFOOD TAHINI SAUCE

4 tablespoons tahini

Juice of ½ lemon

1 teaspoon garlic powder

1 teaspoon moringa powder, optional

Sea salt and pepper to taste

TAKE out an oven rack and line it with parchment paper. Preheat the oven to 400°F.

SPREAD the potatoes, carrots, and beets over the paper-lined oven rack, return the rack to the oven, and roast for 10 minutes.

ADD the remaining vegetables and chickpeas. Sprinkle with Italian herbs and salt and pepper. Roast for another 15 to 20 minutes, until all the veggies are soft.

IN the meantime, mix together the sauce ingredients in a glass jar. Add water to thin if needed for a creamy sauce. Serve the veggies on a plate, drizzled with the tahini sauce.

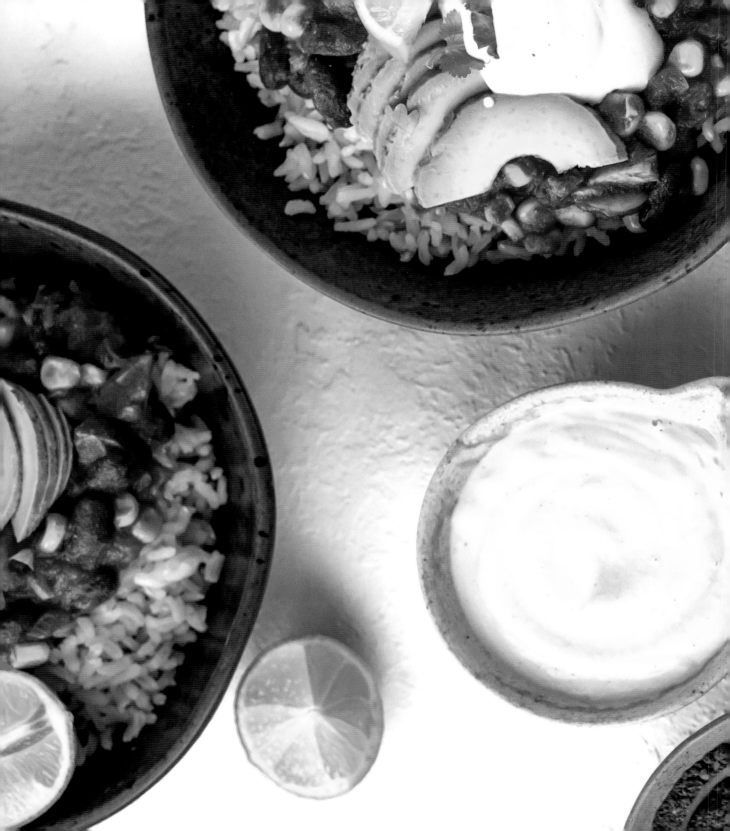

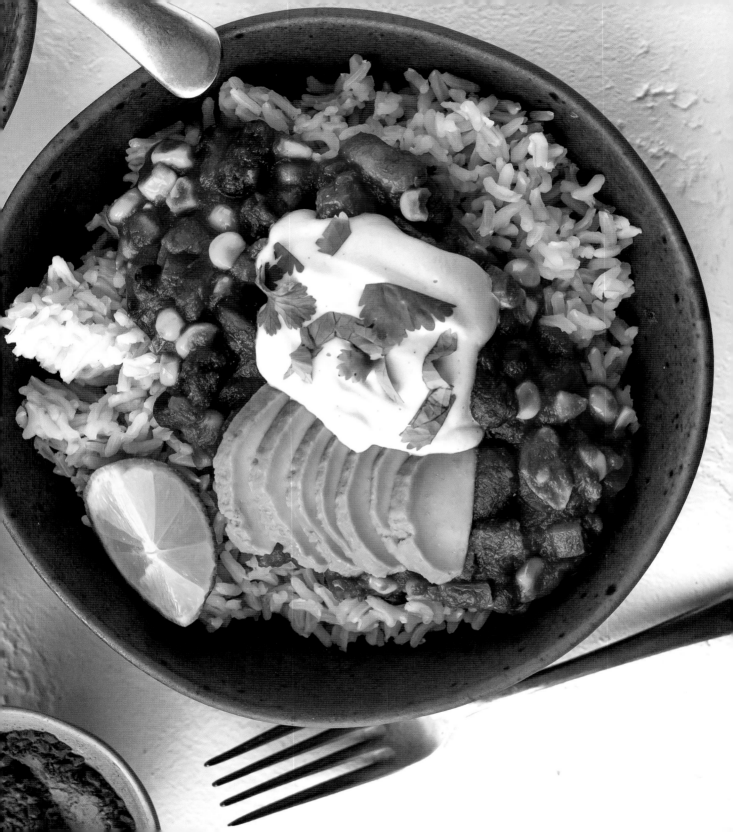

MEXICAN-INSPIRED CHILI BOWL
STRESS REDUCTION

SERVES 2 • This is a chili bowl to chill out with. Reishi is easy to hide in your dinner dishes to help you wind down from the day. This dish comes together quickly, especially if you batch-cook rice or potatoes a couple of times a week so you have those always ready to go—they often take more time than the actual dish. Top with cashew cream and other toppings, if desired..

1 cup brown rice

1 red onion, diced

1 cup sliced button mushrooms

2 cups frozen corn

½ cup tomato paste

2 tomatoes, diced

1 can (15 ounces) kidney beans, about 1½ cups, drained and rinsed

2 teaspoons chili powder

1 teaspoon cumin powder

1 teaspoon garlic powder

2 teaspoons reishi powder, optional

2 teaspoons sriracha sauce

Sea salt and pepper, to taste

CASHEW CREAM (OPTIONAL)

1 cup cashews

½ cup water

1 teaspoon garlic powder

Juice of ½ lime

Pinch of salt

TOPPINGS (OPTIONAL)

½ avocado, sliced

¼ onion, diced

¼ cup diced cilantro

1 tablespoon nutritional yeast

COOK the rice according to the package instructions.

IN a large ceramic-coated frying pan place 1 cup water, the onion, and mushrooms and cook over high heat for 5 minutes.

ADD the corn, tomato paste, tomato, kidney beans, chili powder, cumin, garlic powder, reishi, sriracha, and 1 more cup of water. Stir everything together well; lower the heat to medium and cook for another 10 minutes, stirring occasionally. Remove from heat when it's nice and thick.

TO make the cashew cream, blend all the ingredients in a blender or food processor until smooth and creamy.

SERVE the chili on top of the rice, topped with cashew cream, if desired. Add your favorite toppings.

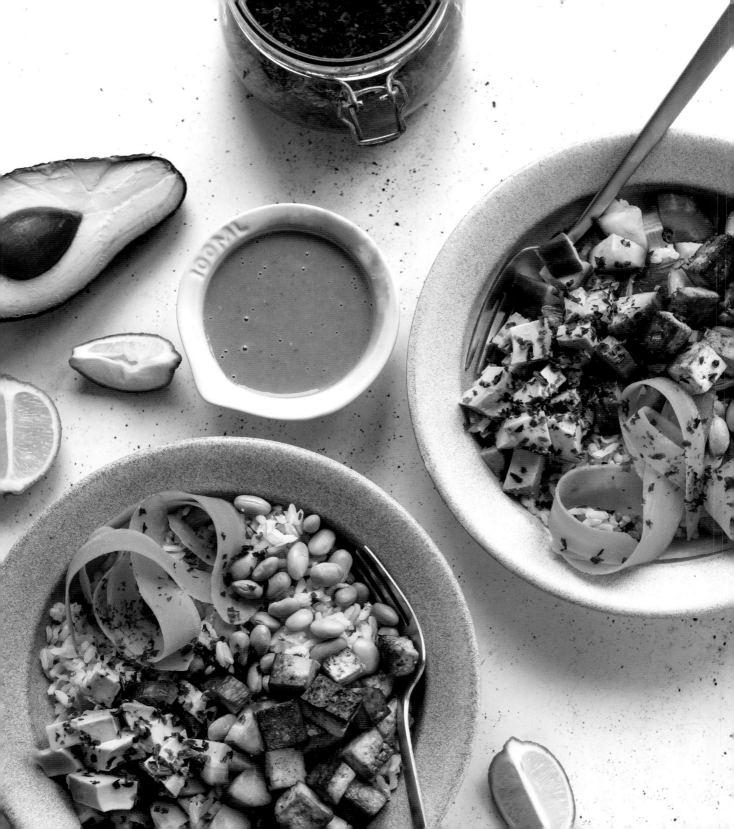

PLANT POWER BOWL
DETOX

SERVES 2 • Nori and kelp are both sea vegetables and true superfoods. They are naturally loaded with iodine, a mineral most of us need more of to support a healthy thyroid. The thyroid gland controls and releases hormones for energy production, growth, and cellular repair. This refreshing dinner features cooked and raw veggies and draws inspiration from Thai cuisine.

1 cup brown rice

1 cup frozen edamame beans

1 tablespoon coconut oil

12 ounces firm tofu, drained, pressed, and cubed

3 tablespoons tamari sauce

PEANUT SAUCE

3 tablespoons peanut butter

1 tablespoon tamari sauce

½ teaspoon chili powder

1 avocado, pitted and cubed

2 carrots, peeled and shredded

¼ cucumber, diced

5 stalks cilantro, optional

1 teaspoon nori or kelp flakes or powder, optional

Juice of ½ lime

Sea salt and pepper to taste

COOK the brown rice according to the package directions, but cook it a little longer than recommended to make a stickier rice, which is nice for this bowl.

STEAM the frozen edamame beans for 5 minutes in ½ inch of water in a pan (or use a basket over boiling water).

PREHEAT a large pan over high heat, add the coconut oil, tofu, and 3 tablespoons tamari sauce. Stir and sauté for 3 to 5 minutes.

STIR the dressing ingredients together in a glass until creamy and thin enough to pour.

TO serve, scoop rice into bowls and top it with the avocado, carrot, cucumber, edamame beans, tofu, and cilantro, if using. Sprinkle nori or kelp flakes or powder on top, if using. Drizzle the peanut dressing over the bowl.

LENTIL STEW
HORMONE HEALTH & PLANT PROTEIN

SERVES 2 • Humble lentils are powerhouses of nutrition. Lentils are actually edible seeds from the legume family. There are many types of lentils, most commonly: brown, puy, green, yellow, red, and beluga. Lentils are made up of more than 25 percent protein. They're also a great source of iron and fiber, which supports regular bowel movements and the growth of healthy gut bacteria. Lentils also contain health-promoting polyphenols, which have strong antioxidant and anti-inflammatory properties with potential cancer cell–inhibiting effects. Here we add health-promoting maca in our twist on this classic comfort food.

1½ cups red lentils, rinsed

½ leek, white and green parts, diced

1 carrot, diced

1 red bell pepper, seeded and diced

1 onion, diced

3 garlic cloves, peeled

3 potatoes, diced

3 teaspoons cumin

2 teaspoons chili powder

3 teaspoons maca powder, optional

2 tablespoons nutritional yeast, optional

Sea salt and pepper to taste

ADD 4 cups of water to a large pot over medium-high heat. Add all the ingredients to the pot and bring to a boil.

TURN down the heat, cover, and simmer for 40 minutes, or until the potatoes are soft when pierced with a fork. Add more water if needed.

TO serve, ladle into 2 bowls and enjoy warm.

VEGGIE MELANZANE
IMMUNITY

SERVES 2 • This is our twist on an Italian dish that originated in the southern regions of Campania and Sicily. We made it vegan and added a bigger variety of veggies, but didn't skimp on what makes it delicious: perfectly cooked eggplant for that umami taste in a delightfully seasoned sauce. We love this dusted with nutritional yeast, but to make it extra special you can also add vegan cashew cheese, vegan mozzarella, or vegan feta on top. Keep some fresh basil to use as garnish just before serving.

1 eggplant, sliced

1 onion, sliced

3 tomatoes, sliced

2 portobello mushrooms, sliced

1 zucchini, sliced

½ cup fresh basil, cut into small strips

1 teaspoon tulsi powder, optional

Sea salt and pepper, to taste

4 cups tomato sauce

5 tablespoons nutritional yeast, optional

2 tablespoons oregano powder

PREHEAT the oven to 400°F.

IN a 9x13-inch oven-safe dish, layer all the veggies on top of each other.

STIR basil, tulsi, salt, and pepper into the tomato sauce. Pour the sauce over the veggies, making sure the veggies are 80 percent covered by the sauce.

ADD the nutritional yeast, if using, and oregano on top and bake for 40 to 45 minutes until all the veggies are cooked.

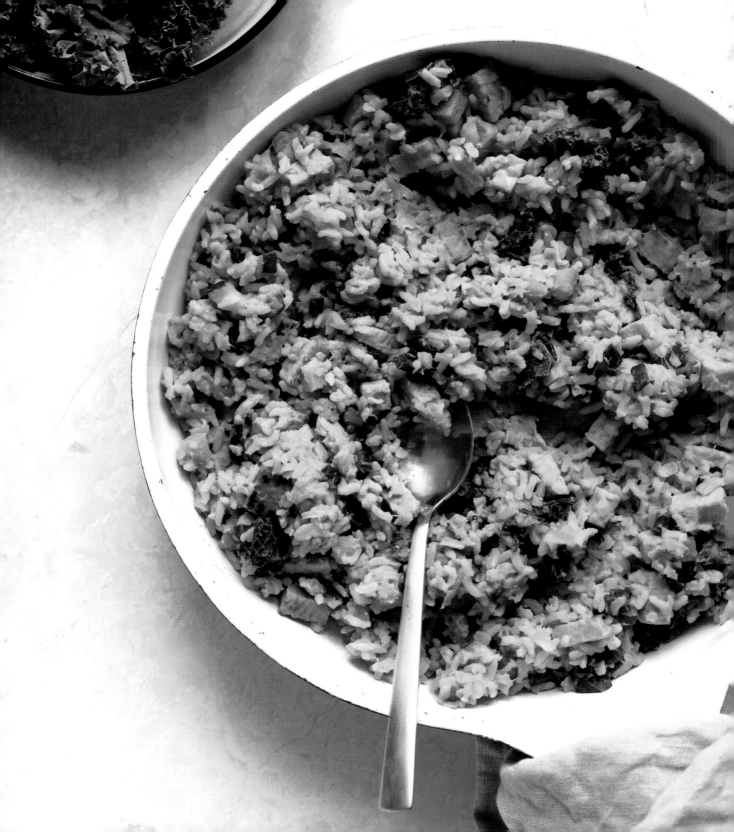

FRIED VEGGIE RICE
DETOX

SERVES 2 • Though tempeh isn't quite as popular as tofu, it is a mainstay of many vegetarian and vegan diets. It's made by fermenting cooked soybeans and then forming the mixture into a firm, dense cake. The fermentation gives tempeh an earthy, savory, mushroom-like flavor and chewy structure. It tends to absorb the flavors of any sauce or spices to which it is added, making it a versatile choice for many sorts of dishes!

2 tablespoons coconut oil

1 white onion, diced

2 garlic cloves, peeled and minced

1 cup pumpkin or squash, diced

1 zucchini, diced

1 cup tempeh, diced

2 cups leftover cooked brown rice

2 cups kale, destemmed and chopped

PEANUT BUTTER SAUCE

4 tablespoons peanut butter

½ cup canned coconut milk

2 teaspoons tamari

1 teaspoon chili powder

1 teaspoon spirulina powder, optional

Sea salt and pepper to taste

MELT the coconut oil in a large ceramic-coated frying pan over high heat. Add the onion and garlic and sauté for two minutes.

ADD pumpkin and 1 cup of water, lower the heat, and simmer for 10 to 15 minutes. Add the zucchini and tempeh and cook for another 5 minutes. Add the cooked brown rice and kale and cook for 3 minutes until the rice is warm and the kale is steamed.

COMBINE the sauce ingredients in a glass jar or mug and mix with a fork. Add about three-quarters of the sauce to the stir-fry and gently toss until evenly distributed.

ENJOY as is or serve with the additional peanut butter sauce.

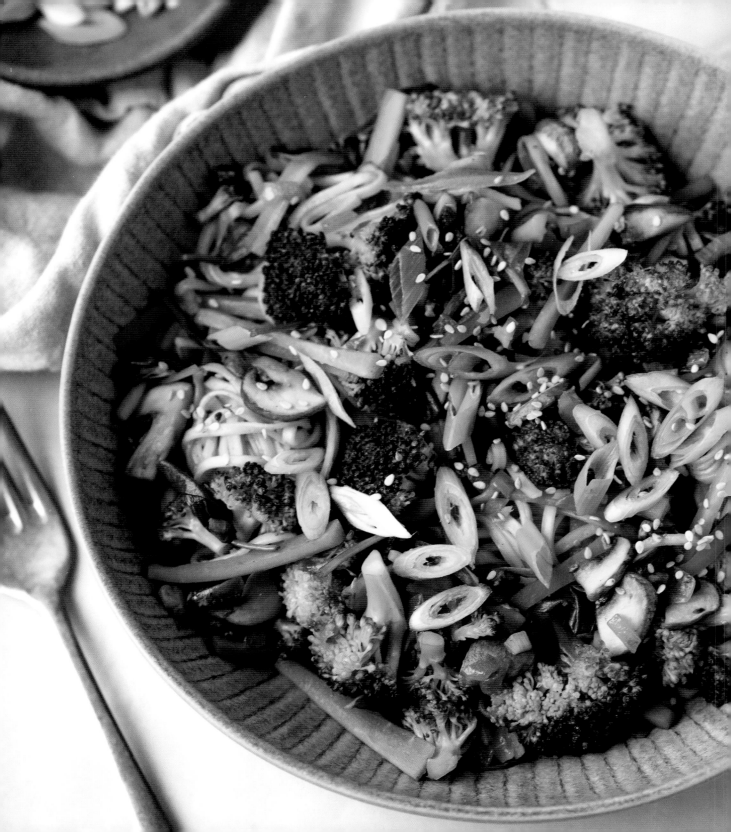

STIR-FRY NOODLES
IMMUNITY & STRESS REDUCTION

SERVES 2 • This easy and delicious dish hits the spot every time. Don't stress if you don't have broccoli, mushrooms, and spinach on hand—just use whatever you have. Rice or buckwheat noodles can be found in the Asian food aisle in most grocery stores, or try an Asian food market. They cook quickly and are naturally gluten-free. Any of the mushroom superfood powders, such as reishi, are a great addition to this dish for an extra boost of added immunity.

8-ounce package rice or buckwheat noodles

1 tablespoon coconut oil

1 white onion, diced

2 garlic cloves, peeled and minced

4 scallions, sliced

1 inch ginger root, minced

1 carrot, sliced

3 cups white button mushrooms, sliced

6 ounces firm tofu, drained, pressed, and cubed, optional

5 tablespoons tamari

Pepper to taste

1 cup spinach, rinsed

1 cup broccoli florets

1 teaspoon reishi powder, optional

Sesame seeds, optional

COOK the noodles according to the package instructions. You want to slightly undercook them, because you will still stir-fry them for an additional 3 to 5 minutes.

HEAT the coconut oil in a ceramic-coated stir-fry pan over high heat. Add the onion, garlic, scallions, and ginger and sauté until the onions are translucent, about 2 minutes.

ADD the carrots and mushrooms to the pan and continue stir-frying for a few minutes. Check the noodles for doneness; drain and set aside. Add tofu to the stir fry, along with tamari and pepper to taste.

ADD the spinach, broccoli, and cooked noodles and stir-fry for another 3 to 5 minutes before removing from the heat. Add reishi powder at the last minute to stir through, if using. Add more tamari if you like. Garnish with more scallions and sesame seeds, if using.

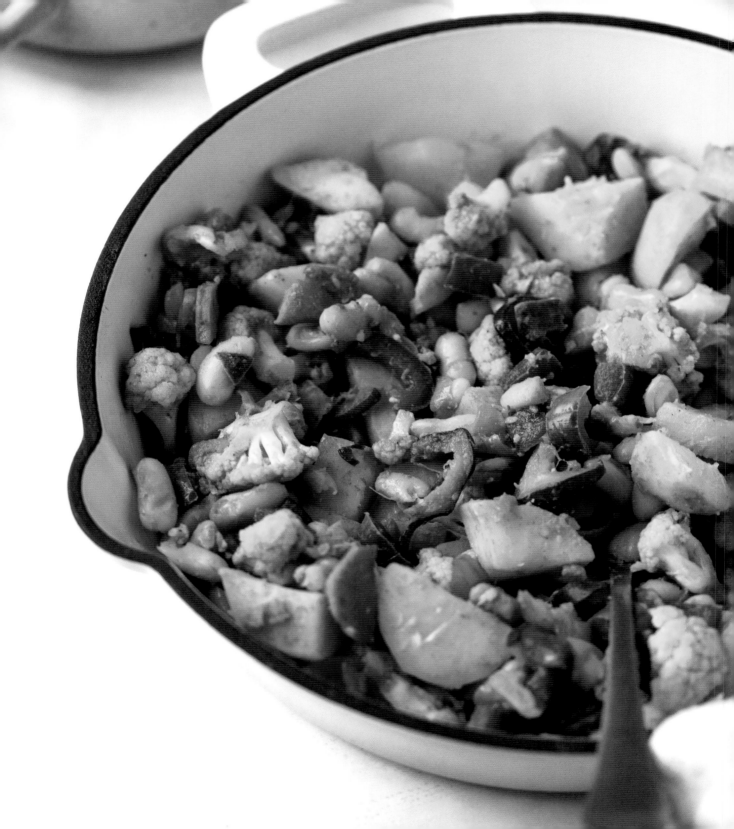

INDIAN-INSPIRED STIR-FRY
IMMUNITY & ANTI-INFLAMMATORY

SERVES 2 • This spicy dish is full of Ayurvedic herbs. Ayurveda, or Ayurvedic medicine, is a healthy-lifestyle system that people in India have used for more than 5,000 years. It emphasizes the prevention and treatment of illness through lifestyle practices and herbal remedies. Any type of white beans will work—great northern, navy, or cannellini beans are good options.

2 tablespoons coconut oil

2 inches fresh ginger root, minced

1 onion, diced

4 garlic cloves, peeled and minced

1 carrot, diced

½ head cauliflower, chopped

1 green bell pepper, diced

½ zucchini, diced

1 can (15 ounces) great northern white beans, about 1½ cups, drained and rinsed

2 cups cubed, roasted potatoes

2 tablespoons curry powder

1 teaspoon cumin powder

1 teaspoon turmeric powder

1 teaspoon tulsi powder, optional

Sea salt and pepper to taste

YOGURT DIP (OPTIONAL)

2 cups unsweetened coconut, soy, oat, or almond yogurt

¼ cucumber, grated

¼ onion, grated

1 teaspoon cumin

Sea salt to taste

ADD the coconut oil to a large ceramic-coated frying pan over high heat. Add the ginger, onion, and garlic and cook, stirring occasionally, for 2 minutes.

ADD the carrot and cauliflower and stir-fry for 10 minutes. Then add the green bell pepper and zucchini and stir-fry for another 10 minutes.

ADD the beans, potatoes, curry powder, cumin, turmeric, tulsi, if using, salt and pepper and stir-fry for another 5 to 10 minutes depending how soft you like your veggies.

STIR all the ingredients of the yogurt dip together before drizzling over your stir-fry, if using.

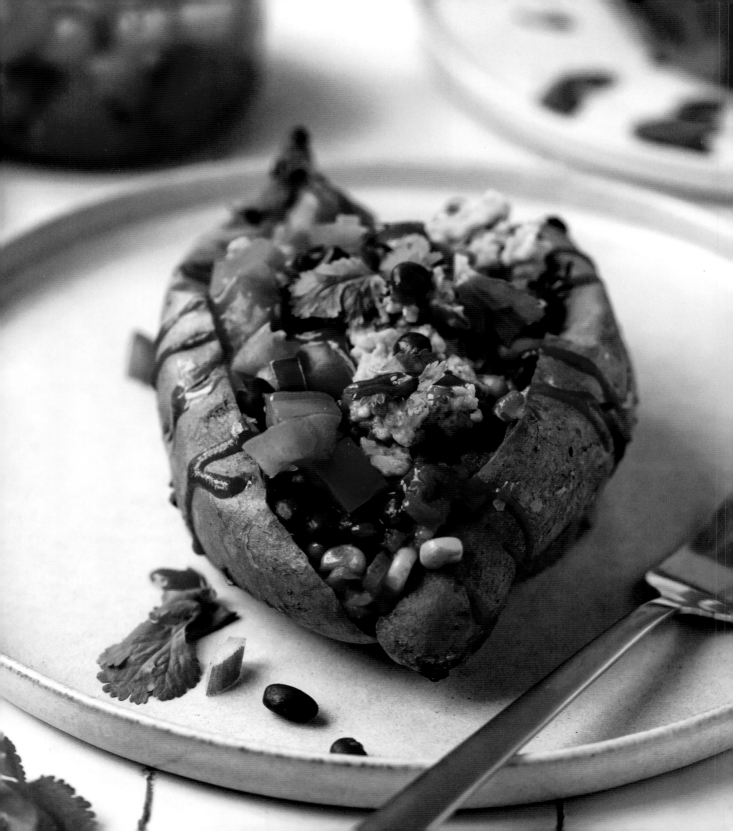

STUFFED SWEET POTATO
DETOX & PLANT PROTEIN

SERVES 2 • This is one of Kristel's favorite recipes—she loves creamy sweet potatoes. Sweet potatoes are starchy root vegetables rich in fiber, vitamin A, vitamin C, manganese, vitamin B_6, potassium, copper, pantothenic acid, and niacin as well as antioxidants that protect your body from free radicals. They also happen to be delicious and versatile. Try our toppings here or experiment with whatever your heart desires!

2 large sweet potatoes

2 tomatoes, diced

1 onion, diced

1 cup frozen corn

¼ cup tomato paste

½ teaspoon chili powder

1 teaspoon wheatgrass powder, optional

Sea salt and pepper to taste

1 avocado, pitted

4 stalks fresh cilantro, roughly chopped

1 can (15 ounces) black beans, about 1½ cups, drained and rinsed

2 tablespoons sriracha sauce

PREHEAT the oven to 400°F. Wash the sweet potatoes, stick some holes on top with a fork, and place in the oven for 30 to 40 minutes until soft.

WHILE your sweet potatoes bake, combine the tomatoes and about half of the onion in a small bowl and mix into a salsa. Set aside.

IN a small pan, combine the rest of the onion, the corn, tomato paste, and ¼ cup of water. Season with the chili powder and wheatgrass, if using, and salt and pepper, to taste. Sauté for 5 to 10 minutes until warm.

IN a small bowl, combine the avocado flesh with the cilantro and more salt and pepper to taste. Mash together with a fork.

TO serve, slice each sweet potato down the middle. Add half of the beans, half of the corn mixture, half of salsa, and mashed avocado on top of each. Top with sriracha sauce.

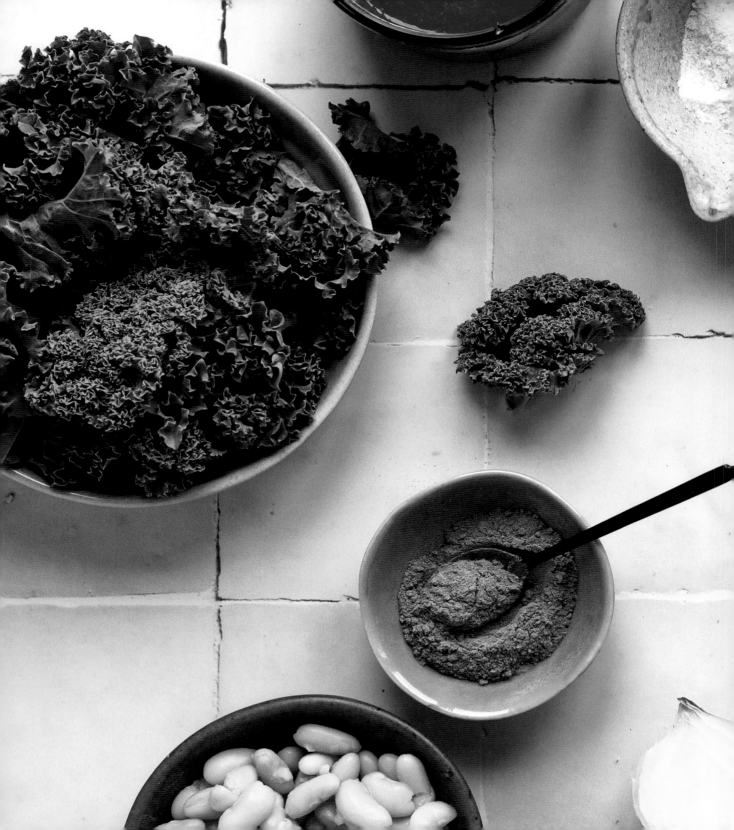

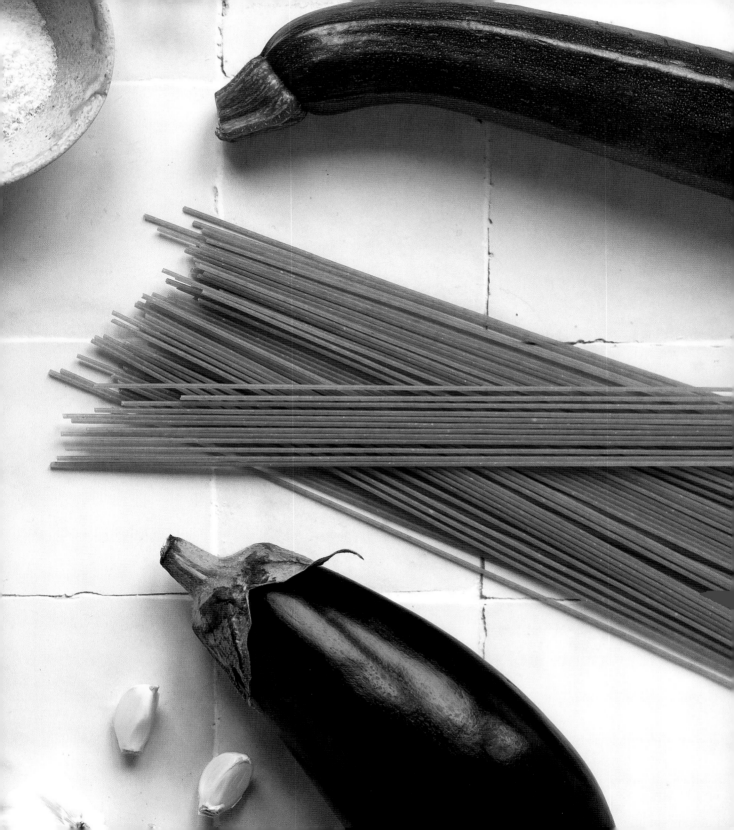

HOW TO MAKE A PASTA BOWL

Pasta gets a bad rap these days, but if done right pasta can be quite healthy and filling, not to mention super easy to make. We love having a quick and easy pasta bowl for dinner. The first secret is to use whole grain pasta instead of pasta made from highly processed wheat flour, which can spike your blood sugar levels. We love gluten-free pasta because we feel it's easier to digest. The second secret is to add a whole bunch of healthy veggies to your tomato sauce. The end result is a beautiful, rich veggie dish that's comforting and filling.

① CHOOSE YOUR GLUTEN-FREE PASTA

Legume, rice, buckwheat, corn, or quinoa are great choices.

② CREATE A BASE OF TOMATO PASTE AND WATER

Create a base by adding tomato paste and water. The ratio of water to tomato paste will depend on how thick or thin you like your tomato sauce. You can also add jarred tomato sauce if you like.

③ CHOOSE TWO OR THREE VEGGIES

For example, eggplant, tomatoes, broccoli, zucchini, mushrooms, kale, onions, or spinach.

④ EXTRAS

For a creamier sauce, add tahini or coconut milk. For a more flavorful sauce, add capers, olives, sun-dried tomatoes, oregano, basil, garlic, pepper, salt, chili, or cayenne powder.

⑤ OPTIONAL

When done cooking, add some extra protein or greens, like chickpeas, tofu, pea protein powder, or super greens like wheatgrass or moringa powder.

TIPS

IF you don't feel like tomato sauce, you can also use a vegan pesto, some olive oil, or a homemade cashew cheese sauce (blend ¼ cup cashews with ¼ cup water, 3 tablespoons nutritional yeast, and salt and pepper to taste).

SPRINKLE with nutritional yeast or vegan parmesan if desired.

WE love combining pasta with a fresh salad for a complete meal. Simply grab a bowl and throw in some greens and your favorite vegetable with noodles and a quick sauce.

IF you have a spiralizer, you can also make pasta with zucchini ("zoodles") or another vegetable like sweet potato (just sauté this for 2 to 3 minutes to cook before eating).

IF you prefer to make your own tomato sauce, blend 4 or 5 tomatoes with herbs, spices, salt and pepper.

HOW TO MAKE A VEGGIE STIR-FRY

Healthy, delicious, and super easy to make, we love veggie stir-fries. There are endless combinations you can try so it never gets boring. Follow these simple steps:

① HEAT THE PAN

Melt one tablespoon of coconut oil in a large ceramic-coated frying pan or use water.

② CHOOSE YOUR VEGGIES

- 3 to 5 minutes for spinach, kale, broccoli, avocado, or fresh herbs like cilantro or basil
- 5 to 10 minutes for mushrooms, zucchini, red bell peppers, garlic, onions, or asparagus
- 5 to 10 minutes for tofu, tempeh, chickpeas, or other beans for extra protein
- 5 to 20 minutes for eggplant, carrots, pumpkin, or cauliflower

③ ADD EXTRA FLAVOR

While stirring occasionally, spice it up with pepper, salt, chili, cayenne, oregano, paprika, onion, garlic, basil, or thyme. Optionally, add soy sauce or tamari, tahini, or miso paste, or sprinkle your favorite superfoods on top.

TIPS

SERVE with rice, quinoa, or any other grain on the side. A side salad is also a great option.

NEED more creaminess? Serve with your favorite dressing or dip (see Easy Green Salad dressing on page 137, Tempeh Wrap sauce on page 145, and Thai peanut dressing on page 163 for ideas).

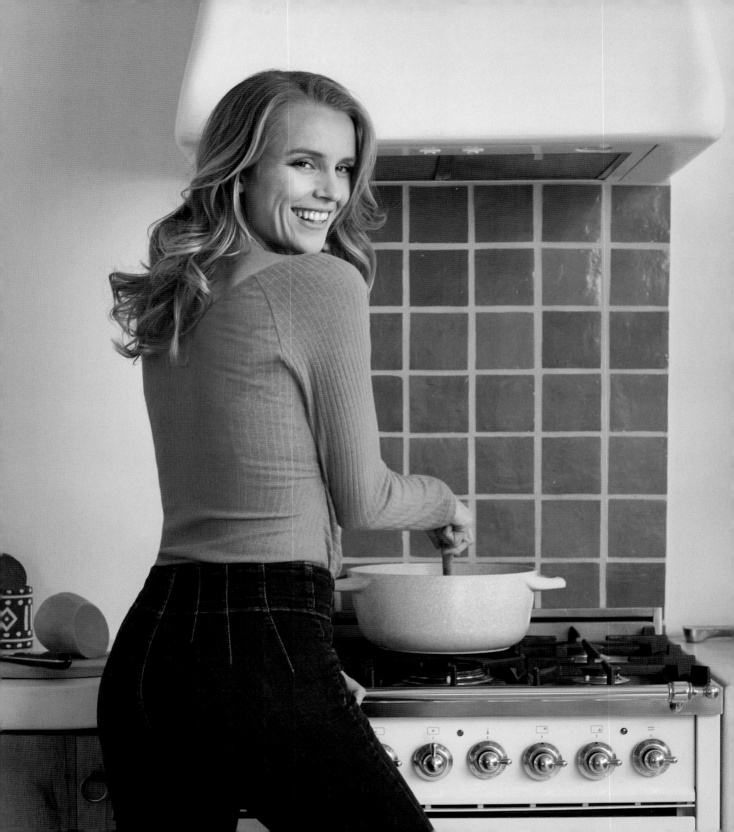

HOW TO MAKE A QUICK CURRY

Curries are our go-to dinners when it's cold. Here's our basic recipe for this popular comfort food. As you can see, curries are very easy to make and really versatile—you can easily mix it up with your favorite veggies.

① THE SAUCE

The curry sauce is made with a 14-ounce can of coconut milk.

② CREAMY VEGGIES

Choose 2 to 3 cups of one base vegetable that will thicken up your curry: sweet potatoes, red lentils, pumpkin, squash, or potatoes.

③ MORE VEGGIES

Choose 2 to 3 cups of additional veggies: eggplant, broccoli, zucchini, mushrooms, kale, onions, spinach, or cauliflower.

④ SPICE IT UP

Add 2 to 4 teaspoons of curry powder and salt and pepper to taste. For extra flavor try adding garlic, onions, chili powder, cayenne, ginger, or turmeric powder.

⑤ EXTRAS

Optional: Top it off with some tahini, fresh herbs, or superfood powders.

TIPS

DON'T have a base veggie on hand, but still craving curry? Go for it! The curry will still taste delicious, the sauce will just be a bit thinner.

YOU can find curry powder mixes in any supermarket. Check the ingredients list for added sugars or other additives.

BLEND your leftover curry with a bit of water or plant milk for a quick and delicious soup!

TOO spicy or not enough flavor? You may want to reduce or increase the amount of curry powder you use. Start with less; you can always add more.

NOURISH

HOW TO MAKE ROASTED VEGGIES

Roasted veggies are another all-time fave of ours. It really doesn't get easier than this and they're so incredibly delicious. Follow these simple steps:

① CHOOSE YOUR VEGGIES

Our favorites include sweet potatoes, pumpkin, broccoli, potatoes, mushrooms, carrots, zucchini, beets, parsnips, brussels sprouts, or onions.

② ROAST IN THE OVEN

Take out an oven rack and line it with parchment paper. Preheat the oven at 400°F. Place the veggies on the parchment paper–covered rack according to approximate cooking time and roast in the oven until crisp:

- 20 to 25 minutes for mushrooms, brussels sprouts, onion, zucchini, broccoli, or asparagus
- 30 to 45 minutes for parsnips, sweet potatoes, potatoes, pumpkin, carrots, or beets

③ ADD YOUR DIPS

Serve with your favorite dips and a side of salad!

TIPS

MAKE more than you need so you have leftovers to add to your lunch bowl the next day.

SPICE it up with salt, pepper, herbs, chili flakes, etc.

SOME people like to roast their vegetables in oil; however, we find that roasting them without oil is super tasty.

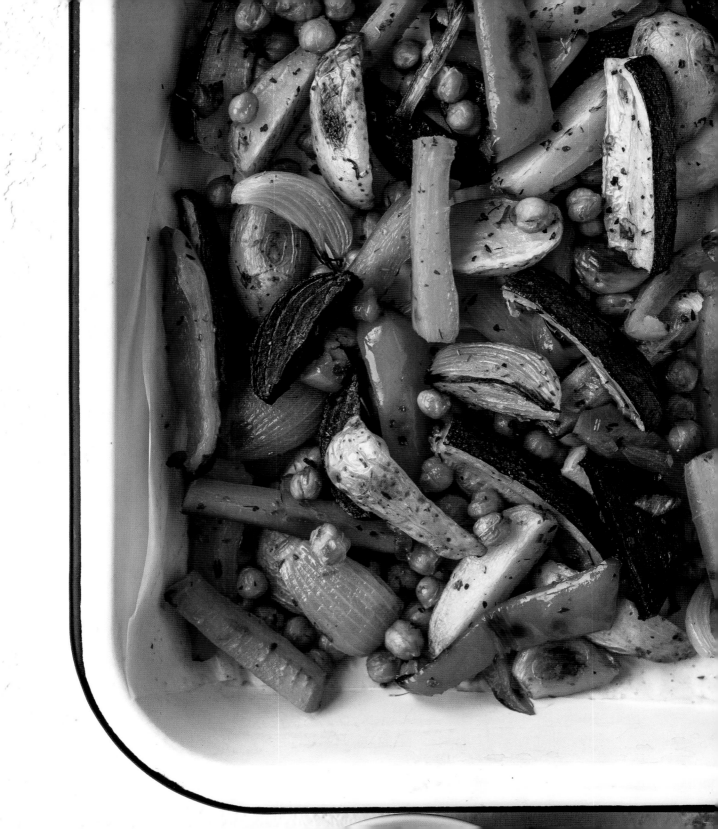

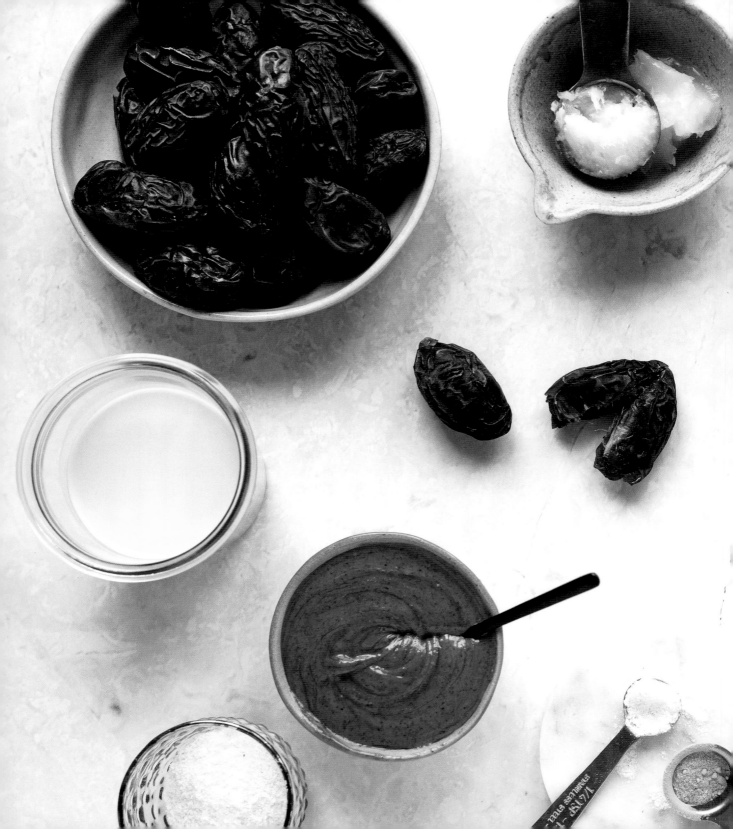

COMFORT
SOUL-SUSTAINING SWEETS

Our favorite sweet things are real, whole foods, as minimally processed as possible—fruit, dates, maple syrup, coconut sugar, and adaptogens and superfoods that nourish and delight us from head to toe. The ingredients in these recipes contain plenty of essential nutrients that take care of your body while you treat yourself—so you get an extra boost of comfort and relaxation at the end of the day.

How many times have you indulged in a decadent dessert only to feel bloated, painfully full, and lethargic just a few minutes after enjoying the last bite? By the way, guilt is a form of stress and can be responsible for some of the not-so-great symptoms we experience after eating something unhealthy. We'll help you fall in love with sweets (all over again), let go of the guilt, and customize your treats with superfoods that support your needs so you can end the day on a sweet note.

You will find plenty of indulgent recipes with cacao as well as specific superfoods that are great at night to calm down, reduce stress, and sleep better. Ashwagandha, tulsi, and reishi feature prominently in this chapter. They all support the body with stress management and calming down so you can sleep better and have more energy the next day.

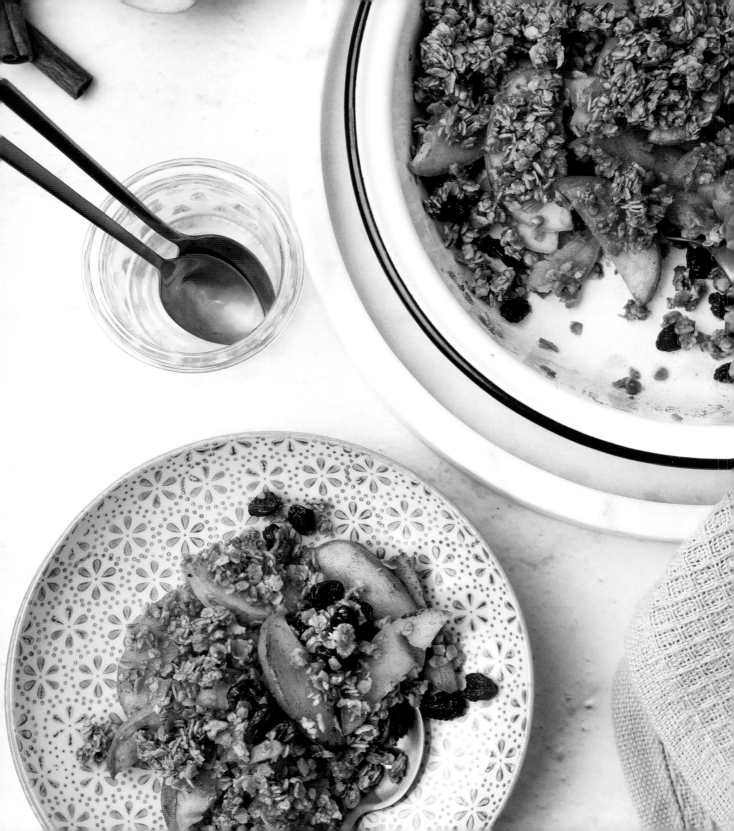

APPLE PROTEIN CRUMBLE
PLANT PROTEIN

SERVES 4 • An apple crumble that's so healthy you can have it for breakfast and so delicious it can be dessert, especially when topped with vegan vanilla ice cream and/or a drizzle of almond butter. We added plant protein to keep you full longer and help balance your blood sugar, and warming cinnamon for anti-inflammatory properties. Pea protein is made by extracting protein from yellow peas. The pea shell is removed and the pea is then milled. It's a great source of protein, containing all nine of the essential amino acids.

APPLE MIXTURE

3 apples, diced

⅓ cup raisins

2 teaspoons cinnamon powder

CRUST

1 cup quick oats

2 tablespoons coconut sugar, optional

2 tablespoons pea protein powder

¼ cup chopped walnuts, optional

PREHEAT the oven to 350°F.

PLACE the apples, raisins, and cinnamon in an oven-safe dish and mix well.

IN a medium-size bowl, place the oats, coconut sugar, if using, pea protein powder, walnuts, if using, with ⅓ cup of water, and mix well until thick and smooth.

POUR crumble mixture over the apples and raisins and bake for 30 minutes or until golden brown.

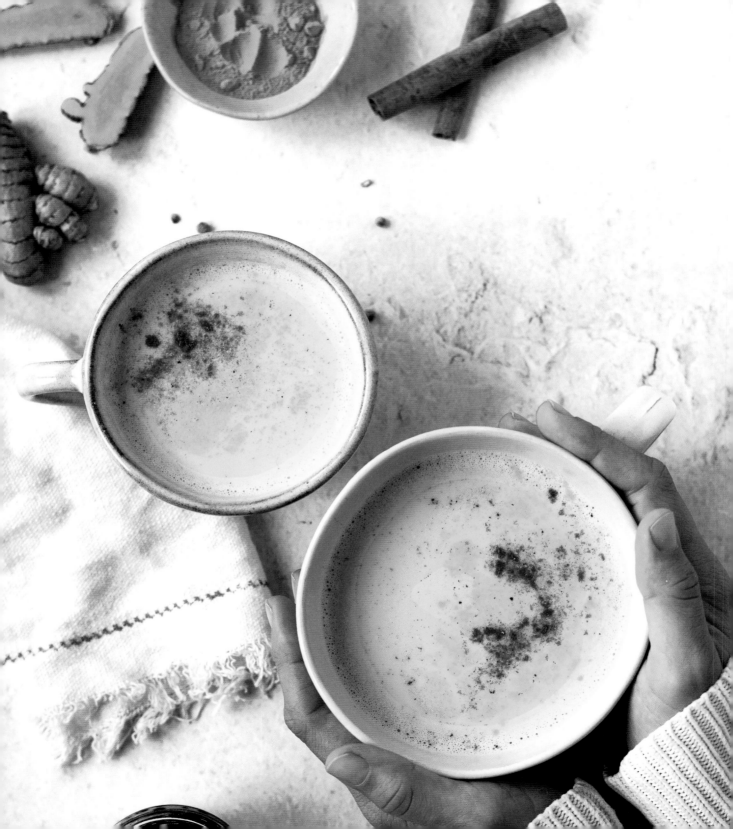

RELAXING TURMERIC LATTE

ANTI-INFLAMMATORY & STRESS REDUCTION

SERVES 2 • A classic turmeric latte is the perfect way to unwind at the end of your day. Tulsi, which is popular in Hindu traditions in India, is an adaptogen that helps calm your nervous system and reduces stress. We love using oat milk in this recipe, but try your favorite plant milk, and be sure to read the ingredient label to find one without sugar, gums, and fillers.

3 cups plant milk

1½ teaspoons turmeric powder

½ teaspoon cinnamon

½ teaspoon tulsi powder, optional

1 teaspoon maple syrup, optional

Sprinkle of pepper

HEAT the milk in a saucepan over medium-low heat.

ADD the turmeric, cinnamon, tulsi, if using, maple syrup, if using, and pepper.

BLEND or use a frother to combine. Enjoy warm.

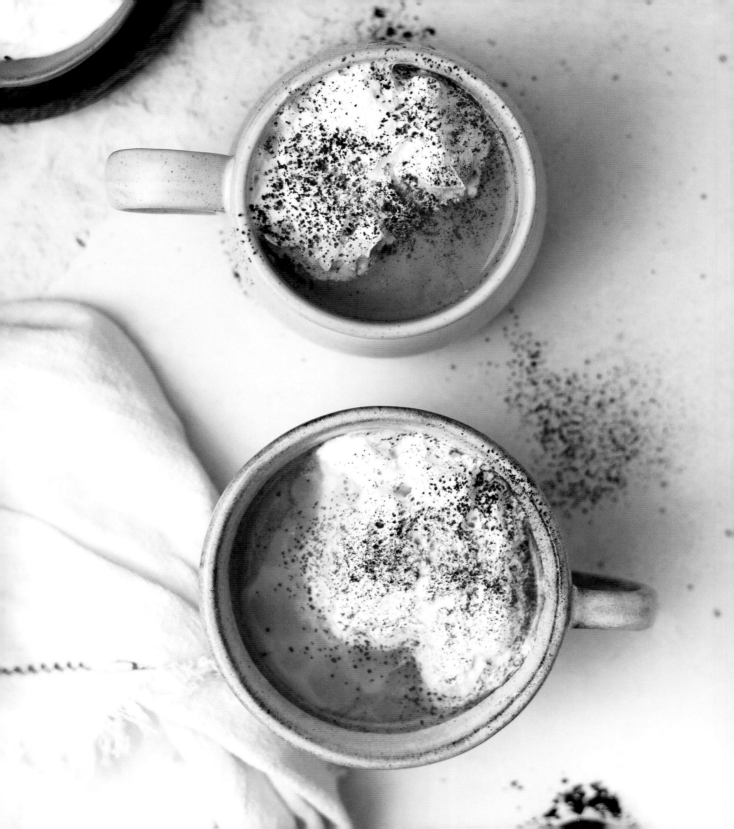

CALMING CHOCOLATE LATTE
STRESS REDUCTION & MOOD BOOSTER

SERVES 2 • A hot chocolate with benefits! Ashwagandha and reishi make this the ultimate evening chill-out drink. The reishi mushroom was first discovered by Chinese healers more than 2,000 years ago in the Changbai Mountains. Native to Europe, Asia, and North America, reishi has been revered in China for thousands of years. Reishi has been used to help enhance the immune system, reduce stress, improve sleep, help you fall asleep faster, and lessen fatigue. This is delicious topped with coconut cream.

3 cups plant milk

2 teaspoons cacao powder

½ teaspoon reishi powder, optional

½ teaspoon ashwagandha powder, optional

½ teaspoon cinnamon powder

1 teaspoon maple syrup, optional

Dollop of coconut cream, optional

STORE a can of coconut milk in the fridge overnight and scoop only the cream from the top, if using.

HEAT the milk in a small saucepan over low to medium heat.

ADD the cacao, reishi, ashwagandha, cinnamon, and maple syrup, if using, and either blend with a spoon or use a frother to combine. Enjoy warm, topped with coconut cream, if desired.

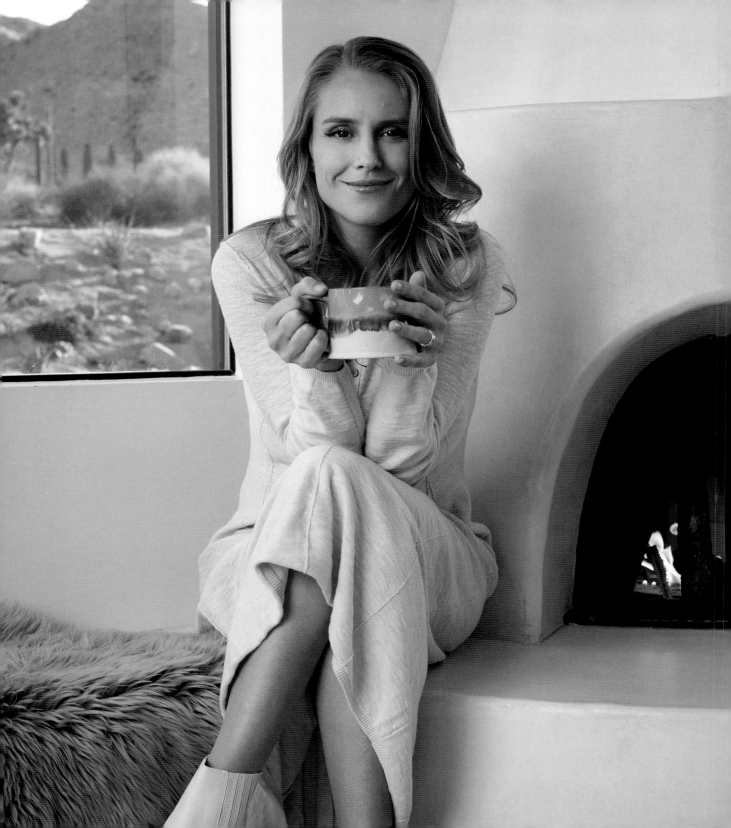

HOMEMADE IMMUNITY TEA

IMMUNITY & ANTI-INFLAMMATORY

SERVES 2 • Kristel prefers brewing her own tea with turmeric and ginger root rather than using tea bags. Homemade tea makes less waste and you can add superfoods that are powerful and delicious. Stock up on fresh ginger and turmeric at home so you have it around whenever you need something warm and soothing before bed. You can reuse the same pieces of ginger and turmeric 3 or 4 times. Besides boosting your immune system, ginger may also alleviate the symptoms of a cold, soothe mild nausea and morning sickness, calm the digestive system, and support heart health.

1 inch fresh ginger root, sliced
1 inch fresh turmeric rhizome, sliced

2 slices lemon or orange, optional

BOIL the ginger, turmeric, and citrus slices, if using, in 3 cups of water for 5 or 10 minutes. Enjoy.

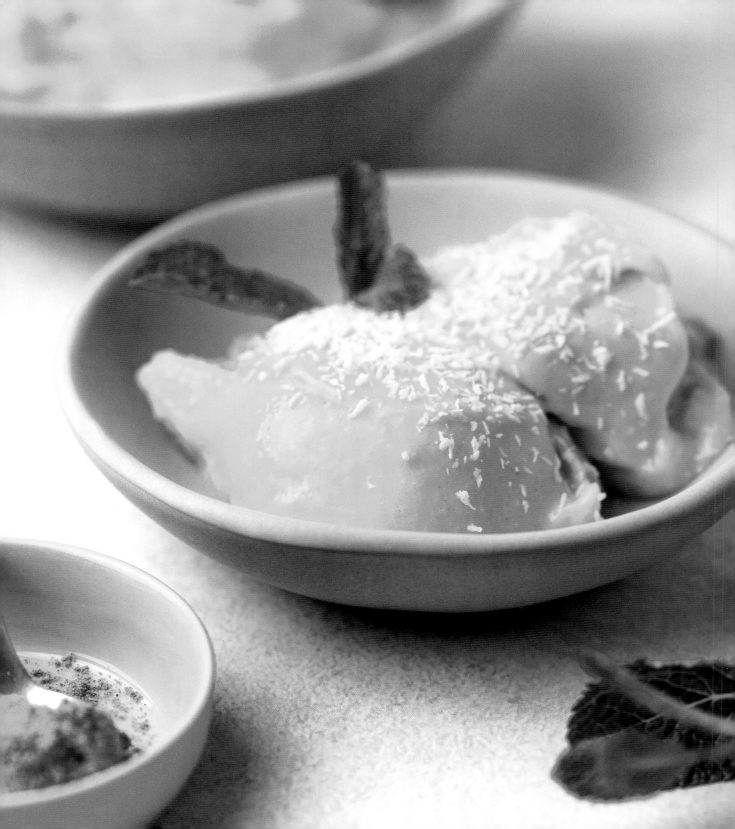

TROPICAL ICE CREAM
IMMUNITY & ANTI-INFLAMMATORY

2 SERVINGS • If you've got frozen fruit stocked in your freezer, you can whip this dessert up in no time. Turmeric helps fight inflammation and the acerola cherry is super high in vitamin C to support your immunity—vitamin C is a powerful antioxidant that protects the body against oxidative stress. Acerola has been found to have up to 14.6 milligrams vitamin C per 1 gram of ripe fruit, which is substantially higher than in other common fruits.

1 cup frozen mango

1 teaspoon turmeric powder

1 teaspoon acerola powder, optional

½ cup unsweetened coconut yogurt or milk

BLEND all the ingredients in a high-speed blender until creamy and smooth.

SERVE plain or with your favorite toppings. Keep leftovers in the freezer.

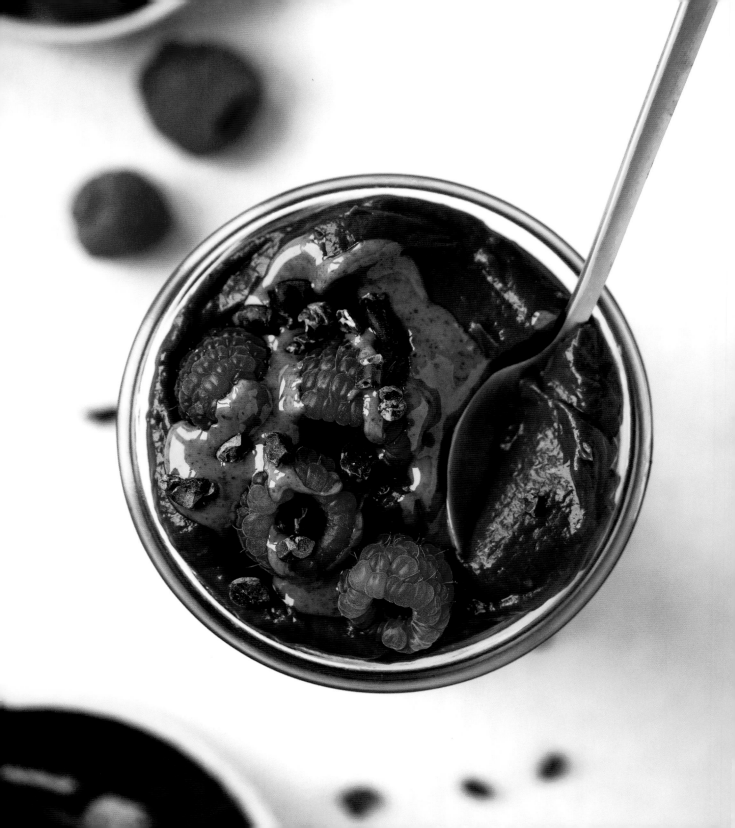

HEALTHY CHOCOLATE MOUSSE
STRESS REDUCTION & MOOD BOOSTER

SERVES 2 • Decadent, rich, filling, and so creamy—and to think you are eating a healthy, green avocado! Most of the healthy fat in avocados is oleic acid, a monounsaturated fatty acid. This heart-healthy fat helps lower cardiovascular inflammation. Avocados also contain a nutrient called beta-sitosterol, the plant version of cholesterol. Beta-sitosterol helps lower your cholesterol levels. You could swap the avocado with a banana if you don't have one on hand or want something sweeter. Top with fresh fruit and your favorite nut butter!

2 tablespoons coconut cream

4 tablespoons cacao powder

½ teaspoon reishi powder, optional

1 ripe avocado

3 tablespoons maple syrup

2 tablespoons almond butter, optional

Pinch of sea salt

STORE a can of coconut milk in the fridge overnight and scoop only the cream from the top.

COMBINE all the ingredients in a high-speed blender or food processor and blend until smooth and creamy.

CHILL in the freezer for 15 minutes to cool down quickly, and serve cold! Store in an airtight container in the fridge for up to 2 days.

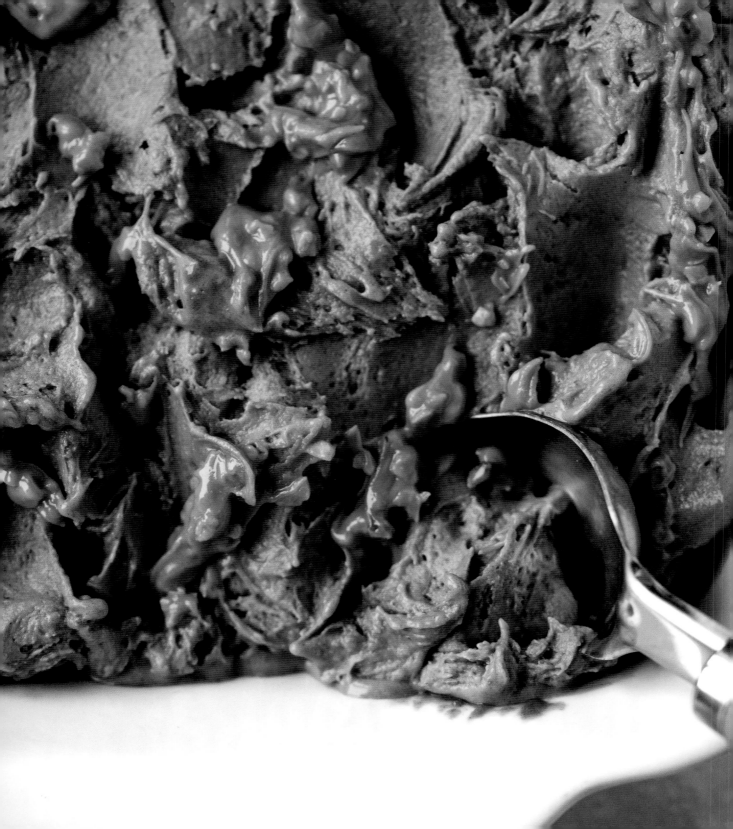

NICE CREAM
STRESS REDUCTION & MOOD BOOSTER

SERVES 2 • I have to warn you that this ice cream is addictively good. If you freeze a banana until solid then whip it up in a blender or food processor, it gets creamy and a little gooey, just like custard ice cream. Bananas are rich in sleep-promoting nutrients like magnesium, tryptophan, vitamin B_6, potassium, and carbs. We love to add a swirl of peanut butter and sprinkle cacao nibs on top.

1 tablespoon peanut butter, plus extra to swirl on top

2 tablespoons cacao powder

½ teaspoon ashwagandha powder, optional

2 teaspoons tocos powder, optional

2 frozen ripe bananas

¼ cup canned coconut milk

Pinch of sea salt

2 tablespoons of cacao nibs, optional

COMBINE all ingredients in a high-speed blender or food processor until smooth.

SCOOP into bowls and top with cacao nibs and peanut butter, if desired. Best eaten immediately.

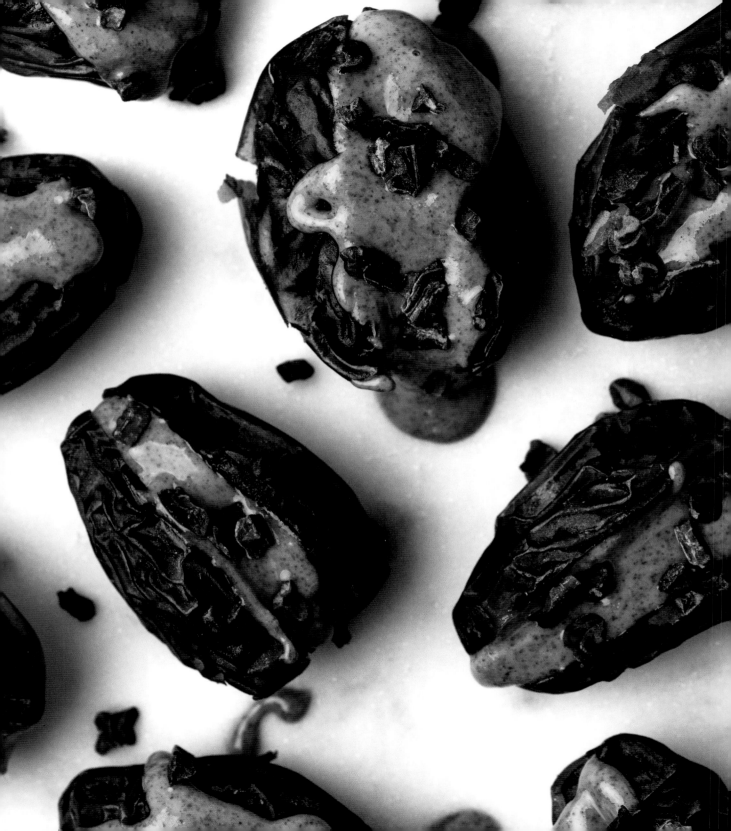

CREAMY CHOCOLATE DATES
MOOD BOOSTER

SERVES 2 • Why do we love cacao? What keeps us coming back for more? It all comes down to the fact that cacao contains a compound called PEA (phenethylamine), which triggers the release of endorphins and mood-enhancing neurochemicals in the brain. Cacao also contains serotonin and tryptophan. Both of these chemicals have been linked to reduced symptoms of depression. In short, cacao makes you feel good. These chocolate dates are perfect to prep in bulk and enjoy through the week. You can also stir turmeric or ginger powder into your almond butter for a little spicy kick and boost of anti-inflammatory health benefits! Look for a one- or two-ingredient almond butter to avoid fillers, sugars, and preservatives. Either salted or unsalted works.

2 tablespoons almond butter

4 pitted medjool dates

4 teaspoons cacao nibs

USING a spoon, fill the dates with the almond butter.

SPRINKLE the cacao nibs on top and enjoy immediately or store in the fridge in a closed container for 3 to 5 days.

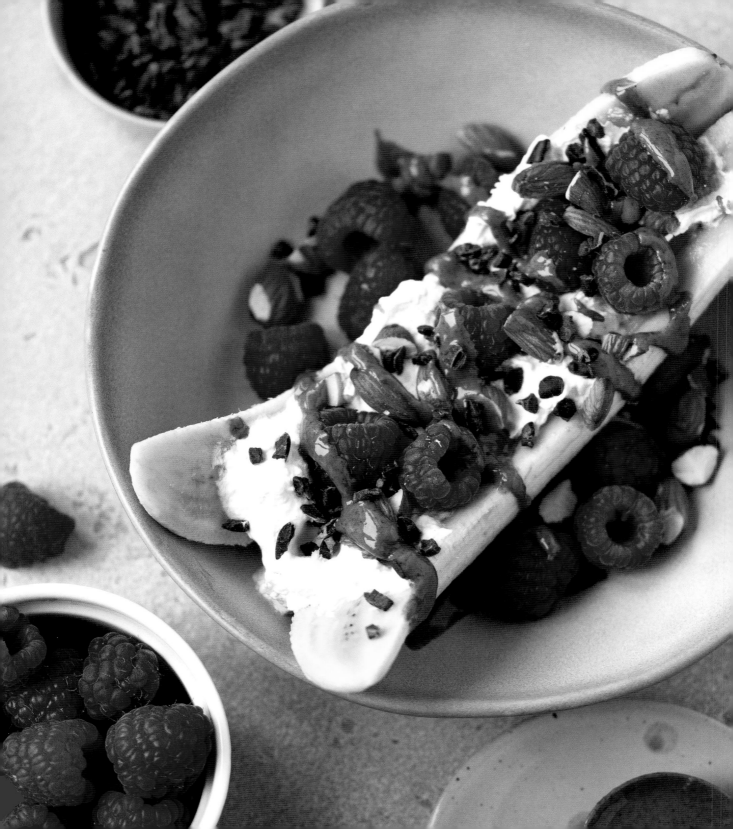

BANANA SPLIT BOWL
MOOD BOOSTER & HEALTHY SKIN

SERVES 1 • This is one of Michael's all-time favorite treats. You simply split a banana and sprinkle everything delicious you can find in your kitchen on top. Go wild and add açaí, maqui powder, or chia seeds, shredded coconut, other nut butters, turmeric powder, or passion fruit. Think of this recipe as a starting point to create your own unique variations. Cacao nibs are small pieces of crushed cacao beans (aka cocoa beans) that have a bitter, chocolatey flavor. Cacao beans are dried after harvesting, then fermented and cracked to produce the small, dark bits—or cacao nibs.

1 banana

3 tablespoons coconut cream

2 tablespoons almonds

2 tablespoons cacao nibs

¼ cup fresh raspberries

1 tablespoon almond butter

STORE a can of coconut milk in the fridge overnight and scoop only the cream from the top.

SLICE the banana lengthwise down the middle. Add the coconut cream on top and spread it across the banana.

CRUSH the almonds into smaller pieces and sprinkle over the banana. Add the remaining toppings—cacao nibs, fresh raspberries, and almond butter—and dive right in!

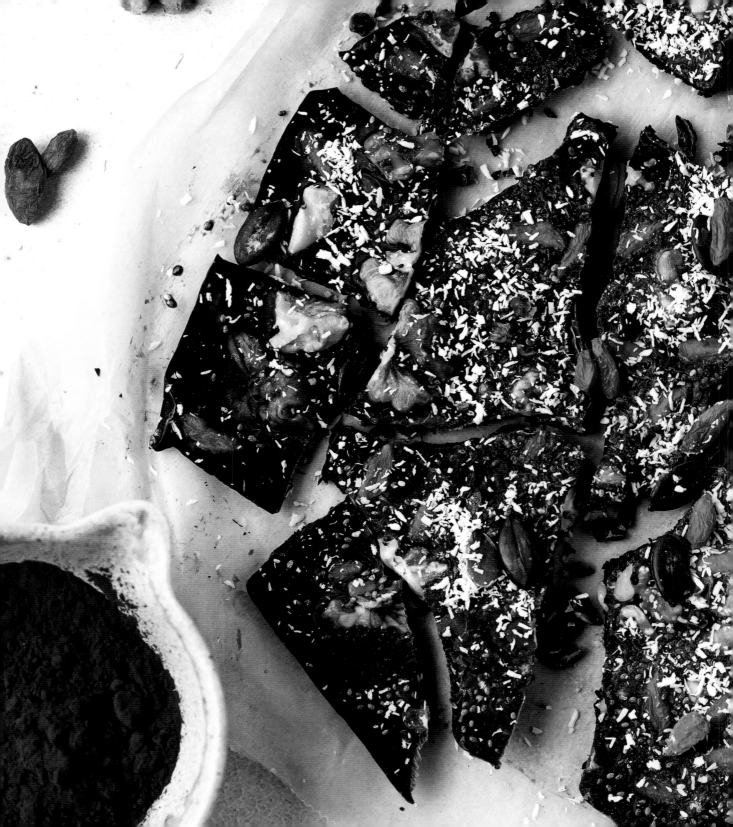

HOMEMADE CHOCOLATE BARK
STRESS REDUCTION & HEALTHY FATS

SERVES 4 • You can get as creative as you want with this recipe by adding different ingredients to the mix, like different dried seeds, almonds, pecans, cashews, dried cherries, goji berries, apricots, or even other powdered superfoods from açaí berries to chaga—whatever extra health benefit you want to add, you name it. Instead of using cacao, coconut oil, and maple syrup you could also melt a vegan dark chocolate bar. Walnuts and chia seeds are packed with omega-3's for a healthy brain and heart!

BASE

½ cup coconut oil

½ cup cacao powder

¼ cup maple syrup

Pinch of sea salt

TOPPINGS

½ cup walnuts, chopped

¼ cup pumpkin seeds

2 teaspoons chia seeds, optional

2 tablespoons shredded coconut

½ cup goji berries, optional

LINE a pan or baking sheet with parchment paper.

IN a medium-size saucepan, melt the coconut oil over low heat.

REMOVE from heat and whisk in the cacao and maple syrup until smooth. Add a pinch of sea salt to taste.

COMBINE all toppings in a separate bowl. Stir in half of the toppings to the chocolate mixture.

WITH a spatula, spoon the chocolate mixture onto the prepared pan or sheet and smooth out until it's ¼ to ½ inch thick. Sprinkle on the remaining toppings. Place in the freezer on a flat surface for about 15 minutes, until frozen solid.

ONCE frozen, break apart into bark. Store in the fridge for 3 to 5 days.

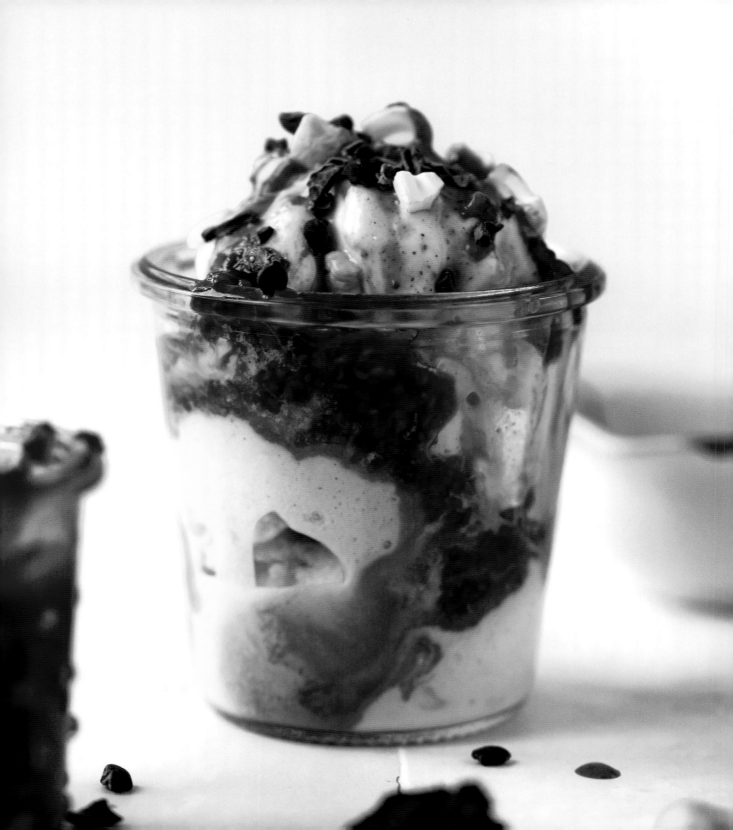

BERRY SUNDAE ICE CREAM

SKIN HEALTH & HEALTHY FATS

SERVES 1 OR 2 • This delicious, easy dessert hits the spot every single time. When buying vanilla vegan ice cream, read the label carefully. Try finding a clean brand without too much gum added to it. If you can't find a vegan ice cream, you can also make your own ice cream base by blending 3 frozen bananas with 2 tablespoons of coconut cream and 1 teaspoon vanilla extract. Maqui and chia seeds are skin-boosting superfoods; you can also add tocos and açaí powder, if desired.

1 cup frozen raspberries

1 teaspoon maqui powder, optional

1 teaspoon chia seeds, optional

3 scoops vanilla plant-based ice cream

2 tablespoons almond butter

1 tablespoon cacao nibs

1 tablespoon broken cashews

IN a saucepan over medium heat, cook the frozen raspberries for about 5 minutes until they are soft and warm. Take the saucepan off the heat and stir in maqui and chia seeds, if using.

PLACE 3 scoops of vanilla ice cream in a bowl (or divide into two if you're sharing).

POUR the raspberry mixture over the ice cream and top it with the almond butter, cacao nibs, and cashews.

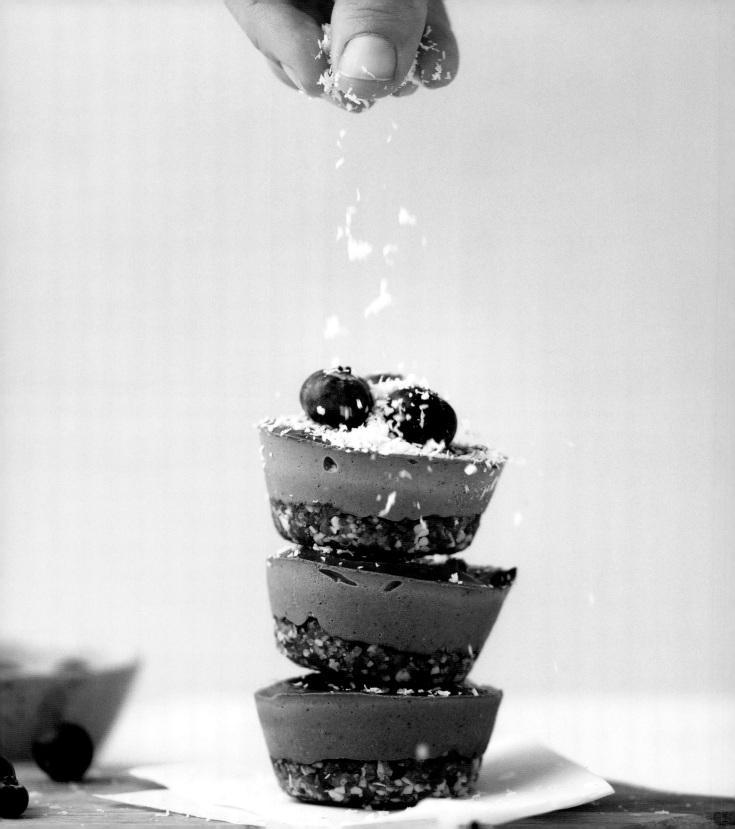

RAW BLUEBERRY CUPCAKES
SKIN HEALTH

SERVES 6 • Berries are a yummy way to improve your overall health, so we eat lots of them. Here, blueberries, açaí berries, and maqui form a trio of powerful antioxidants to protect your body from free radicals, which are unstable molecules that can damage your cells and contribute to aging and diseases, such as cancer. In addition to protecting your cells, these plant compounds may reduce disease risk.

FILLING

1½ cups raw cashews

¼ cup coconut oil

¼ cup plant milk

¼ cup maple syrup

2 tablespoons lemon juice

¼ cup frozen blueberries

2 teaspoons açaí powder

2 teaspoons maqui powder, optional

2 teaspoons tocos powder, optional

BASE

½ cup almonds

1½ cup dates

Pinch of sea salt

SOAK the cashews in hot water for 15 minutes. Drain thoroughly.

MEANWHILE, make the base by blending the almonds, dates, and sea salt in a blender or food processor into a sticky mixture.

LINE a muffin tin with 6 liners or use a silicone muffin pan. Put an equal layer of the almond mixture in the bottom of each liner. Place in the freezer to set.

BLEND all the filling ingredients, including the soaked cashews, together in a high- speed blender or food processor until smooth.

ADD the blueberry filling to the cupcake liners. If you like, top the cupcakes with some frozen berries. Place them back in the freezer for at least an hour. Store in the fridge afterward.

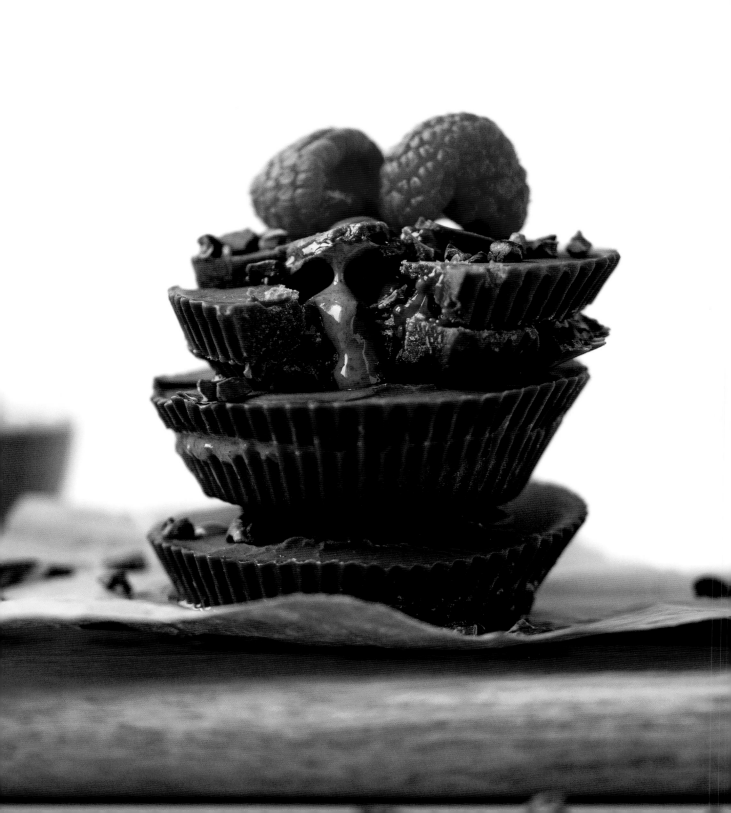

ALMOND BUTTER CUPS
SKIN HEALTH & HEALTHY FATS

SERVES 6 • I often joke that almond butter is the glue that holds my body together. Forget the store-bought peanut butter cups—once you have tried these you will never go back. You can swap almond butter with peanut butter or even tahini if you like. Adding powerful reishi or chaga to the chocolate coating is another great option. The optional berry filling is delicious, so while it's not essential to the recipe, we highly recommend it! This recipe easily doubles if you're using a muffin tin, but I like to use silicone or paper muffin liners and make six just for myself.

8 tablespoons cacao powder

½ cup melted coconut oil

3 tablespoons maple syrup

½ cup almond butter

EXTRA BERRY FILLING (OPTIONAL)

½ cup raspberries

1 tablespoon chia seeds

1 teaspoon açaí powder

1 teaspoon maqui powder

LINE a muffin tin with 6 liners.

IN a bowl, combine the cacao, melted coconut oil, and maple syrup.

SPOON about 2 tablespoons of the chocolate mixture into the muffin liners and freeze for 10 minutes.

ONCE frozen, add a spoonful of the almond butter to the center of each liner. Place back in the freezer.

NOW'S the time to add your berry filling, if using. In a bowl, mix the raspberries, chia seeds, and the açaí and maqui with a fork into one smooth mixture. Add a spoonful of the berry mixture on top of the almond butter in each cup.

SPOON the remaining chocolate mixture over the top of each muffin cup before placing them back into the freezer for 1 hour. Enjoy right away or store in the fridge.

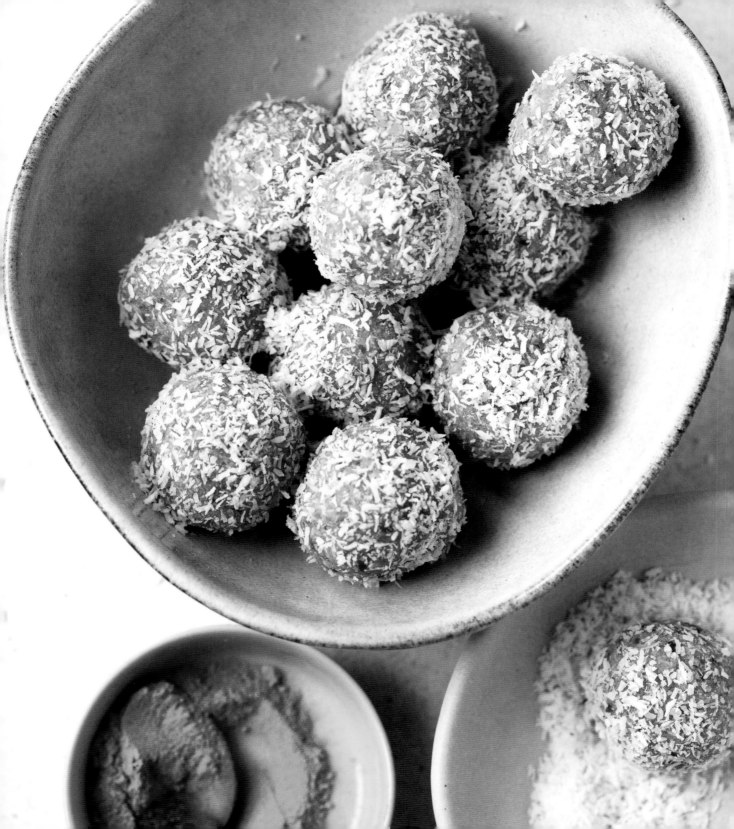

TURMERIC BOUNTY BALLS
ANTI-INFLAMMATORY & STRESS REDUCTION

SERVES 4 • Anti-inflammatory turmeric and calming ashwagandha and tulsi make this the perfect nighttime dessert. Prep a bigger batch so you can have some ready with your favorite evening latte. If you don't like coconut, use cashews instead. Ashwagandha is an adaptogen that can help your body manage stress. It's an ancient medicinal herb used in Ayurveda (just like turmeric) for many years. It also can boost brain function, lower blood sugar and cortisol levels, and help fight symptoms of anxiety and depression. Roll in some leftover shredded coconut for an even more decadent treat.

1½ teaspoons turmeric powder

½ teaspoon ashwagandha powder, optional

½ teaspoon tulsi powder, optional

¾ cup shredded coconut

⅓ cup pitted dates

¼ cup maple syrup

BLEND all the ingredients in a high-speed blender or food processor until sticky. Scrape the sides of the blender if needed.

ROLL into small bite-size balls, about 1½ inches.

STORE in the fridge in an airtight container for 3 to 5 days.

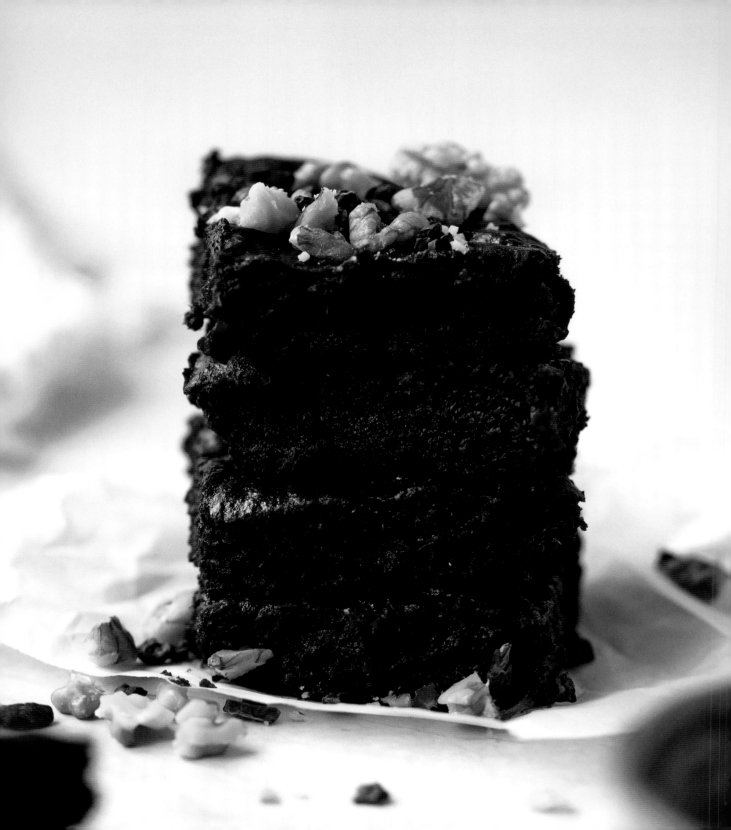

HAPPY BROWNIES
HORMONE HEALTH & MOOD BOOSTER

SERVES 6 • These indulgent brownies are a delicious way to add hormone-balancing superfoods to your day. Maca and shatavari support hormones, fertility, and libido—yes, libido! Maca and shatavari can help you add some spice back into the bedroom. Use these superfoods for 4 to 8 weeks daily to see an improvement.[1] Walnuts and cacao nibs would make great optional toppings. You can also swap the almond butter for tahini or peanut butter if you like.

2 cups pitted dates

1 cup almond flour

¾ cup almond milk

½ cup almond butter

2 tablespoons melted coconut oil

⅓ cup cacao powder

2 teaspoons maca powder, optional

1 teaspoon shatavari powder, optional

Pinch of sea salt

PREHEAT the oven to 350°F and line an 8x8-inch square baking dish with parchment paper.

SOAK the dates in hot water for 5 minutes.

COMBINE all the ingredients in a high-speed blender or food processor and blend until smooth.

ADD the batter to the baking dish and bake for 15 to 20 minutes. Eat warm or cool them and store in the fridge for 3 to 5 days.

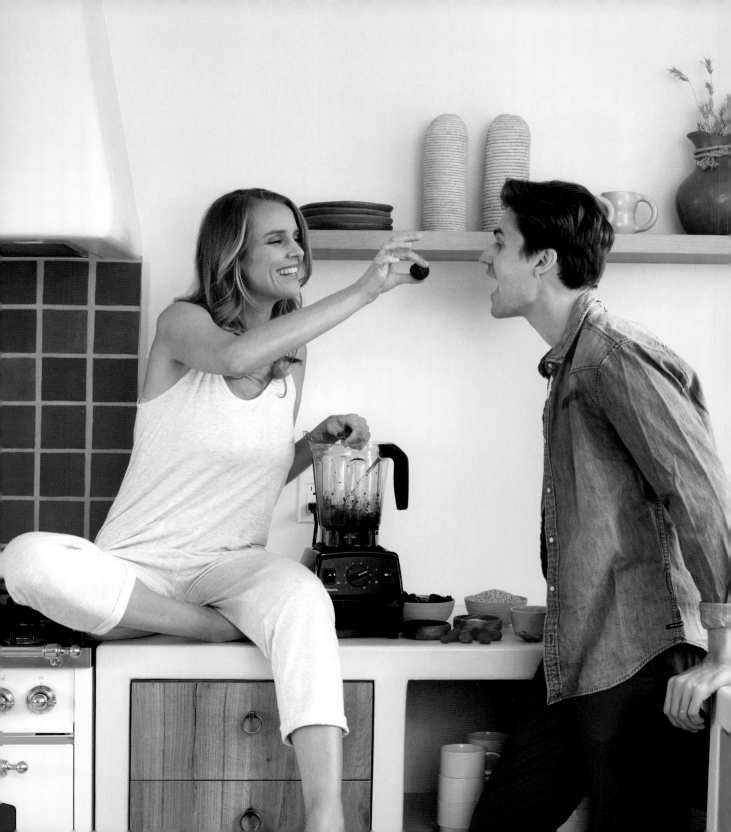

DOUBLE CHOCOLATE BALLS
STRESS REDUCTION & IMMUNITY

SERVES 4 • Chocolate balls dipped in more chocolate . . . Do we need to say more? The filling is perfect to hide some powerful superfoods that will support calming down and better sleep. The chaga mushroom has a host of inspiring health benefits: It enhances the immune system, is a powerful antioxidant, can be used to resolve stomach pain, and has a powerful antiviral action—to name just a few. With its adaptogenic properties, chaga helps your body adapt to stress and calm down after a long day.

FILLING

⅓ cup quick oats

2 teaspoons cacao powder

½ teaspoon ashwagandha powder, optional

½ teaspoon chaga powder, optional

¼ cup peanut butter

¼ cup raisins

BASE

¼ cup coconut oil

¼ cup cacao powder

2 tablespoons maple syrup

Pinch of sea salt

BLEND all the filling ingredients in a high-speed blender or food processor. Roll into small 1½-inch balls, place them on a plate, and store them in the freezer.

IN a medium-size saucepan, melt the coconut oil over low heat. Remove from the heat and whisk in the cacao powder and maple syrup until smooth. Add a pinch of sea salt to taste.

REMOVE the balls from the freezer and dip them into the chocolate sauce. Place back on the plate to store them in the freezer again for about 15 minutes.

ENJOY afterward or store in the fridge in a sealed container for 3 to 5 days.

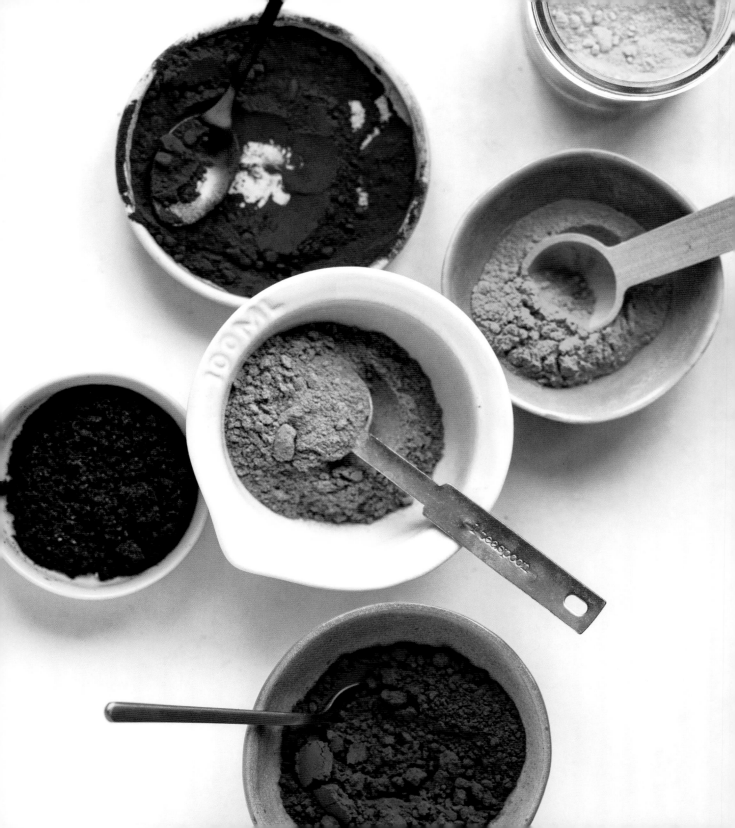

YOUR SUPER MIXES

If you're new to superfoods and not sure where to start, we've highlighted our top 10 superfood powders that we recommend trying first. These mixes are easy to access and have a good variety of different benefits and can be used in many recipes.

1. Açaí
2. Cacao
3. Wheatgrass
4. Turmeric
5. Reishi
6. Pea Protein
7. Chia Seeds
8. Ginger
9. Ashwagandha
10. Maca

You can also buy Your Super mixes on **www.yoursuper.com** instead of buying everything loose. Great mixes to start with that will be easy to use in the recipes in this book are Super Green, Energy Bomb, Forever Beautiful, Golden Mellow, Gut Feeling, Plant Protein, Magic Mushroom, and Skinny Protein. Once you're using these in your daily meals, you can try adding Plant Collagen, Moon Balance, and Gut Restore. If you go this route, use the table below to see which mixes work with each recipe.

CHAPTER 4

BAOBAB LEMONADE: Super Green, Gut Feeling, Gut Restore

SPARKLING TURMERIC REFRESHER: Golden Mellow, Gut Restore

DETOX WATER: Super Green, Gut Feeling

ENERGIZING BERRY WATER: Forever Beautiful, Energy Bomb

SUPERFOOD CRACKERS: Super Green, Gut Feeling

KIDNEY BEAN HUMMUS: Forever Beautiful

GREAT NORTHERN BEAN HUMMUS: Plant Protein, Super Green

ENERGY GUAC: Super Green, Gut Feeling

ROASTED NUTS: Super Green

ROASTED CHICKPEAS: Golden Mellow

GREEN LEAFY CHIPS: Super Green

SUPERFOOD POPCORN: Super Green, Forever Beautiful, Magic Mushroom

POWER CHOCO SMOOTHIE: Magic Mushroom, Plant Protein

SUPER POPS: Super Green, Golden Mellow, Moon Balance, Magic Mushroom

BERRYLICIOUS MILKSHAKE: Forever Beautiful, Plant Collagen

CHAPTER 5

EGGPLANT PASTA: Super Green

EASY TACOS

MEXICAN-INSPIRED CHILI BOWL: Magic Mushroom

MUSHROOM RISOTTO

EASY PUMPKIN CURRY: Golden Mellow

ROASTED RAINBOW VEGGIES: Super Green

CHEESY CAULIFLOWER & FRIES: Golden Mellow

EASY GREEN STIR-FRY: Golden Mellow

FRIED VEGGIE RICE: Super Green

LENTIL STEW

STUFFED SWEET POTATO: Super Green

PLANT POWER BOWL

STIR-FRY NOODLES

VEGGIE MELANZANE: Super Green, Gut Feeling

INDIAN-INSPIRED STIR-FRY: Golden Mellow

CHAPTER 6

APPLE PROTEIN CRUMBLE: Plant Protein

CALMING CHOCOLATE LATTE: Magic Mushroom, Plant Collagen

BANANA SPLIT BOWL: Forever Beautiful, Magic Mushroom

CREAMY CHOCOLATE DATES

NICE CREAM: Magic Mushroom, Plant Collagen

HEALTHY CHOCOLATE MOUSSE: Magic Mushroom

TROPICAL ICE CREAM: Golden Mellow, Gut Restore

HOMEMADE IMMUNITY TEA: Golden Mellow, Gut Restore

RELAXING TURMERIC LATTE: Golden Mellow, Plant Collagen

HOMEMADE CHOCOLATE BARK: Magic Mushroom

BERRY SUNDAE ICE CREAM: Forever Beautiful

RAW BLUEBERRY CUPCAKES: Forever Beautiful, Plant Collagen

ALMOND BUTTER CUPS: Magic Mushroom, Forever Beautiful

TURMERIC BOUNTY BALLS: Golden Mellow

HAPPY BROWNIES: Magaic Mushroom, Plant Protein, Moon Balance

DOUBLE CHOCOLATE BALLS: Magic Mushroom

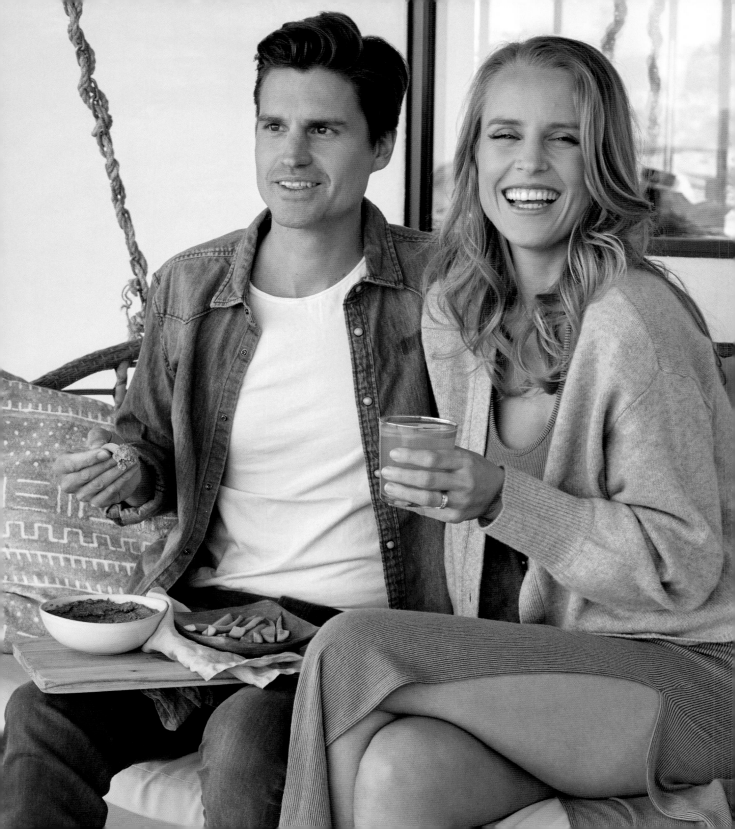

ACKNOWLEDGMENTS

Thank you, Mom, for letting me help you cook when I was little and therefore learned how to cook, combine ingredients, and be creative in the kitchen from such a young age. And for teaching me about the important relationship between what I eat and my health.

We are grateful for Amy who believed in us enough to kick-start this book project and turn it into a reality. Thank you, Stephanie, Colleen, and Sarah for working on this book together for the past year and making it so much better than we ever thought was possible.

Thank you, Patricia, for taste-testing everything, food styling, and shooting the most beautiful, mouth-watering food pictures. And Stefanie, we appreciate you for authentically capturing Michael and me in our natural habitat . . . cooking, laughing, and eating in the kitchen!

A shout-out to all organic farmers around this world, who are so often forgotten, who grow the most healing fruits and vegetables with so much patience and love. Something we all need more of!

And last but not least, we are grateful for the Your Super community who fuel our energy to keep doing what we are doing every day . . . improving people's health with the power of super plants!

XO Kristel & Michael

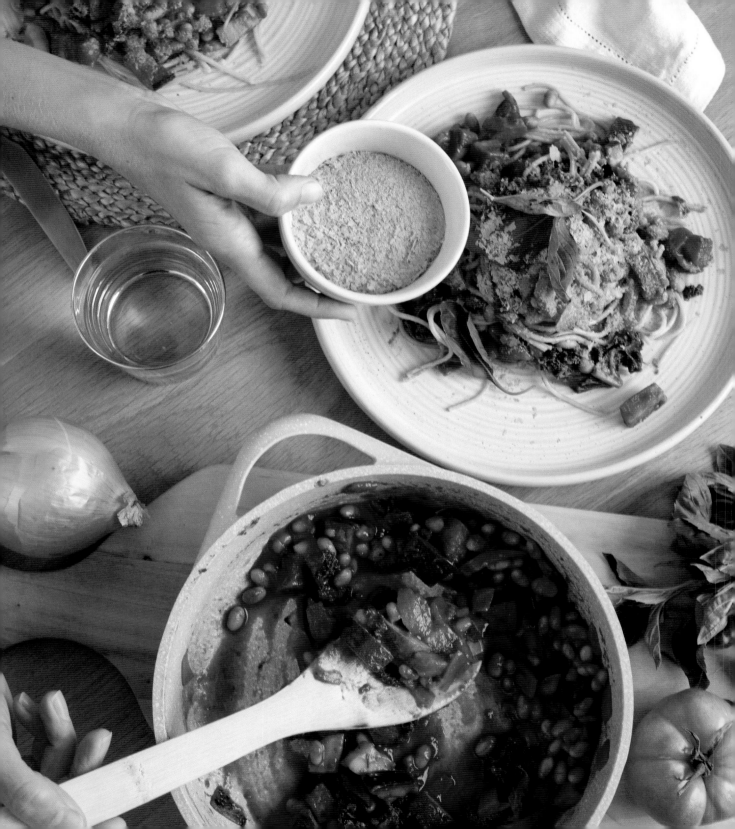

ENDNOTES

Introduction

1. World Health Organization. "Cancer." February 3, 2022. https://www.who.int/news-room/fact-sheets/detail/cancer.
2. World Health Organization. "Diet, Nutrition and the Prevention of Chronic Diseases." 2003. http://apps.who.int/iris/bitstream/handle/10665/42665/WHO_TRS_916.pdf;jsessionid=CDCB15ACD6A249FB309725A3AF548D52?sequence=1.
3. World Health Organization. "Healthy Diet." April 29, 2020. https://www.who.int/news-room/fact-sheets/detail/healthy-diet.
   World Health Organization. "The Top 10 Causes of Death." December 9, 2020. https://www.who.int/news-room/fact-sheets/detail/the-top-10-causes-of-death..
   Fulkerson, Lee, dir. *Forks Over Knives*. Monica Beach Media, 2011. https://www.forksoverknives.com/the-film/.
   Campbell, T. Colin, and Thomas M. Campbell. *The China Study: The Most Comprehensive Study of Nutrition Ever Conducted and the Startling Implications for Diet, Weight Loss, and Long-Term Health*. Dallas: BenBella Books, 2006.

Your Super Way of Eating

1. Madigan, Mariah, and Elisa Karhu. "The Role of Plant-Based Nutrition in Cancer Prevention." *Journal of Unexplored Medical Data* 3, no. 9 (2018). https://doi.org/10.20517/2572-8180.2018.05.
2. Watzl, Bernhard. "Anti-Inflammatory Effects of Plant-Based Foods and of Their Constituents." *International Journal for Vitamin and Nutrition Research* 78, no. 6 (December 2008):293–298. https://pubmed.ncbi.nlm.nih.gov/19685439/.
3. McMacken, Michelle, and Sapana Shah. "A Plant-Based Diet for the Prevention and Treatment of Type 2 Diabetes." *Journal of Geriatric Cardiology* 14, no. 5 (May 2017): 342–354. https://www.ncbi.nlm.nih.gov/pmc/articles/PMC5466941/.

4. Kahleova, Hana, Susan Levin, and Neal D. Barnard. "Vegetarian Dietary Patterns and Cardiovascular Disease." *Progress in Cardiovascular Diseases* 61, no. 1 (May–June 2018): 54–61, https://doi.org/10.1016/j.pcad.2018.05.002.

5. Hope R. Ferdowsian and Neal D. Barnard. "Effects of Plant-Based Diets on Plasma Lipids." *The American Journal of Cardiology* 104, no. 7: 947–956 (October 2009). https://pubmed.ncbi.nlm.nih.gov/19766762/.

6. Jiang, Xian, Jiang Huang, Daqiang Song, Ru Deng, Jicheng Wei, and Zhuo Zhang. "Increased Consumption of Fruit and Vegetables Is Related to a Reduced Risk of Cognitive Impairment and Dementia: Meta-Analysis." *Frontiers in Aging Neuroscience* 9, no. 18 (2017). https://www.frontiersin.org/article/10.3389/fnagi.2017.00018.

7. Tomova, Aleksandra, Igor Bukovsky, Emilie Rembert, Willy Yonas, Jihad Alwarith, Neal. D. Barnard, and Hana Kahleova. "The Effects of Vegetarian and Vegan Diets on Gut Microbiota." *Frontiers in Nutrition* 6, no. 47 (April 2019). https://www.frontiersin.org/articles/10.3389/fnut.2019.00047/full..

8. Barnard, Neal D., David M. Goldman, James F. Loomis, Hana Kahleova, Susan M. Levin, Stephen Neabore, and Travis C. Batts. "Plant-Based Diets for Cardiovascular Safety and Performance in Endurance Sports." *Nutrients* 11, no. 1 (January 2019): 130. https://pubmed.ncbi.nlm.nih.gov/30634559/..

9. Clinton, Chelsea M., Shanley O'Brien, Junwen Law, Colleen M. Renier, and Mary R. Wendt. "Whole-Foods, Plant-Based Diet Alleviates the Symptoms of Osteoarthritis." *Arthritis* 2015 (2015): 708152. https://doi.org/10.1155/2015/708152.

10. Medawar, Evelyn, Sebastian Huhn, Arno Villringer, and A. Veronica Witte. "The Effects of Plant-Based Diets on the Body and the Brain: A Systematic Review." *Translational Psychiatry* 9, no. 226 (2019). https://doi.org/10.1038/s41398-019-0552-0.

11. Kahleova, Hana, Rebecca Fleeman, Adela Hlozkova, Richard Holubkov, and Neal D. Barnard. "A Plant-Based Diet in Overweight Individuals in a 16-Week Randomized Clinical Trial: Metabolic Benefits of Plant Protein." *Nutrition & Diabetes* 8, no. 1 (November 2018):58. https://www.nature.com/articles/s41387-018-0067-4.
Kahleova, Hana, Marta Klementova, Vit Herynek, Antonin Skoch, Stepan Herynek, Martin Hill, Andrea Mari, and Terezie Pelikanova. "The Effect of a Vegetarian vs Conventional Hypocaloric Diabetic Diet on Thigh Adipose Tissue Distribution in Subjects with Type 2 Diabetes: A Randomized Study." *Journal of the American College of Nutrition* 36, no. 5 (364–369). https://doi.org/10.1080/07315724.2017.1302367.

12. Malter, M., G. Schriever, and U. Eilber. "Natural Killer Cells, Vitamins, and Other Blood Components of Vegetarian and Omnivorous Men." *Nutrition & Cancer* 12, no. 3 (1989): 271–278. https://pubmed.ncbi.nlm.nih.gov/2771803/.3.

13. Akbaraly, Tasnime N., Eric J. Brunner, Jane E. Ferrie, Michael G. Marmot, Mika Kivimaki, and Archana Singh-Manoux. "Dietary Pattern and Depressive Symptoms in Middle Age." *British Journal of Psychiatry* 195, no. 5 (2009): 408–413. https://pubmed.ncbi.nlm.nih.gov/19880930/..

14. Malter, M., G. Schriever, and U. Eilber. "Natural Killer Cells, Vitamins, and Other Blood Components of Vegetarian and Omnivorous Men." *Nutrition & Cancer* 12, no. 3 (1989): 271–278. https://pubmed.ncbi.nlm.nih.gov/2771803/.

15. Tanaka, T, K. Kouda, M. Kotani, A. Takeuchi, T. Tabei, Y. Masamoto, H. Nakamura, M. Takigawa, M. Suemura, H. Takeuchi, and M. Kouda. "Vegetarian Diet Ameliorates Symptoms of Atopic Dermatitis Through Reduction of the Number of Peripheral Eosinophils and of PGE2 Synthesis by Monocytes." *Journal of Physiological Anthropology and Applied Human Science* 20, no. 6 (November 2001): 353–361. https://pubmed.ncbi.nlm.nih.gov/11840688/.

16. Centers for Disease Control and Prevention. "Only 1 in 10 Adults Get Enough Fruits or Vegetables." CDC Newsroom. November 16, 2017. https://www.cdc.gov/media/releases/2017/p1116-fruit-vegetable-consumption.html.1.

17. Eurostat. "Fruit and Vegetable Consumption Statistics." Statistics Explained. March 2018. https://www.farmersfresh.eu/wp-content/uploads/2022/03/Fruit-Vegetable-consumption-statistics-in-the-EU.pdf.1.

18. Intergovernmental Panel on Climate Change. "Climate Change and Land: An IPCC Special Report on Climate Change, Desertification, Land Degradation, Sustainable Land Management, Food Security, and Greenhouse Gas Fluxes in Terrestrial Ecosystems." Summary for Policymakers. 2019. https://www.ipcc.ch/srccl/chapter/summary -for-policymakers/.

19. Stancheva, Terry. "50+ Terrifying Factory Faming Facts to Know in 2022." Pawsome Advice. May 2, 2021. https:// pawsomeadvice.com/environment/factory-farming-facts/.

20. Ibid.

21. Xu, Xiaoming, Prateek Sharma, Shijie Shu, Tzu-Shin Lin, Philippe Ciais, Francesco N. Tubiello, Pete Smith, Nelson Campbell, and Atul K. Jain. "Global Greenhouse Gas Emissions from Animal-Based Foods Are Twice Those of Plant-Based Foods." *Nature Food* 2 (2021): 724–732. https://doi.org/10.1038/s43016-021-00358-x.

22. Poore, Joseph, and Thomas Nemecek. "Reducing Food's Environmental Impacts Through Producers and Consumers." *Science* 360, no. 6392 (June 2018): 987–992. https://www.science.org/doi/10.1126/science.aaq0216.

23. Stancheva, Terry. "50+ Terrifying Factory Faming Facts to Know in 2022." Pawsome Advice. May 2, 2021. https:// pawsomeadvice.com/environment/factory-farming-facts/.

24. American Psychological Association. "Stressed in America." *Monitor on Psychology* 42, no. 1 (January 2011): 60. https://www.apa.org/monitor/2011/01/stressed-america.

25. Carrington, Damian. "Chemical Pollution Has Passed Safe Limit for Humanity, Say Scientists." *The Guardian*. January 18, 2022. https://www.theguardian.com/environment/2022/jan/18/chemical-pollution-has-passed-safe -limit-for-humanity-say-scientists.

26. SciNews, "Scientists Categorize Earth as a 'Toxic Planet.'" Phys.org. February 7, 2017. https://phys.org/news/2017 -02-scientists-categorize-earth-toxic-planet.html.

27. Goyal, Ankit, Vivek Sharma, Neelam Upadhyay, Sandeep Gill, and Manvesh Sihag. "Flax and Flaxseed Oil: An Ancient Medicine and Modern Functional Food." *Journal of Food Science and Technology* 51, no. 9 (September 2014): 1633–1653. https://www.ncbi.nlm.nih.gov/pmc/articles/PMC4152533/.

Your Super Life Kitchen

1. Soil Association. "Why Organic?" n.d. https://www.soilassociation.org/take-action/organic-living/why-organic/.

A Last Word on Health

1. Rosenkranz, Melissa A., Richard J. Davidson, Donal G. MacCoon, John F. Sheridan, Ned H. Kalin, and Antoine Lutz. "A Comparison of Mindfulness-Based Stress Reduction and an Active Control in Modulation of Neurogenic Inflammation." *Brain, Behavior, and Immunity* 27 (January 2013): 174–184. https://www.sciencedirect.com/science/ article/abs/pii/S0889159112004758.

2. Orme-Johnson, David W., and Vernon A. Barnes. "Effects of the Transcendental Meditation Technique on Trait Anxiety: A Meta-Analysis of Randomized Controlled Trials." *Journal of Alternative and Complementary Medicine* 20, no. 5 (May 2014): 330–341. https://pubmed.ncbi.nlm.nih.gov/24107199/.

3. Ong, Jason C., Rachel Manber, Zindel Segal, Yinglin Xia, Shauna Shapiro, and James K. Wyatt. "A Randomized Controlled Trial of Mindfulness Meditation for Chronic Insomnia." *Sleep* 37, no. 9 (September 2014): 1553–1563. https://academic.oup.com/sleep/article/37/9/1553/2416992.

4. Bai, Z., J. Chang, C. Chen, P. Li, K. Yang, and I. Chi. "Investigating the Effect of Transcendental Meditation on Blood Pressure: A Systematic Review and Meta-Analysis." *Journal of Human Hypertension* 29, no. 11 (November 2015): 653–662. https://pubmed.ncbi.nlm.nih.gov/25673114/.

5. Norris, Catherine J., Daniel Creem, Reuben Hendler, and Hedy Kober. "Brief Mindfulness Meditation Improves Attention in Novices: Evidence from ERPs and Moderation by Neuroticism." *Frontiers in Human Neuroscience* 12 (2018): 315. https://www.ncbi.nlm.nih.gov/pmc/articles/PMC6088366/.

Chapter 1: Uplift: Build a Better Breakfast

1. American Institute for Cancer Research. "Soy: Intake Does Not Increase Risk for Breast Cancer Survivors." April 8, 2021. https://www.aicr.org/cancer-prevention/food-facts/soy/.
2. He, Fen-Jin, and Jin-Qiang Chen. "Consumption of Soybean, Soy Foods, Soy Isoflavones and Breast Cancer Incidence: Differences Between Chinese Women and Women in Western Countries and Possible Mechanisms." *Food Science and Human Wellness* 2, no. 3–4 (September–December 2013): 146–161. https://www.sciencedirect.com/science/article/pii/S2213453013000438.

Chapter 2: Refresh: Vibrant Midmorning Snacks

1. Meissner, H. O., P. Mrozikiewicz, T. Bobkiewicz-Kozlowska, A. Mscisz, B. Kedzia, A. Lowicka, H. Reich-Bilinska, W. Kapczynski, and I. Barchia. "Hormone-Balancing Effect of Pre-Gelatinized Organic Maca (Lepidium peruvianum Chacon): (I) Biochemical and Pharmacodynamic Study on Maca Using Clinical Laboratory Model on Ovariectomized Rats." *International Journal of Biomedical Science* 2, no. 3 (2006): 260–272. https://www.ncbi.nlm.nih.gov/pmc/articles/PMC3614604/.
2. Breus, Michael J. "Should You Drink Coffee or Matcha for Better Sleep?" *Psychology Today.* July 26, 2019. https://www.psychologytoday.com/us/blog/sleep-newzzz/201907/should-you-drink-coffee-or-matcha-better-sleep.
3. Rahmani, Arshad H., Salah M. Aly, Habeeb Ali, Ali Y. Babiker, Sauda Srikar, and Amjad A. Khan. "Therapeutic Effects of Date Fruits (Phoenix dactylifera) in the Prevention of Diseases via Modulation of Anti-inflammatory, Anti-oxidant and Anti-tumour Activity." *International Journal of Clinical and Experimental Medicine* 7, no. 3 (2014): 483–491. https://www.ncbi.nlm.nih.gov/pmc/articles/PMC3992385/.

Chapter 4: Support: Hunger-Busting Afternoon Snacks

1. McManus, Katherine D. "Should I Be Eating More Fiber?" *Harvard Health Blog.* February 27, 2019. https://www.health.harvard.edu/blog/should-i-be-eating-more-fiber-2019022115927.

Chapter 5: Nourish: Making Dinner a Healing Ritual

1. Asp, Karen. "Why Eat More Mushrooms, Doctors Say: They Boost Immunity and Fight Cancer." The Beet. May 15, 2021. https://thebeet.com/why-eat-more-mushrooms-doctors-say-they-boost-immunity-fight-cancer/?utm_source=tsmclip&.

Chapter 6: Comfort: Soul-Sustaining Sweets

1. Gonzales. G. F., A. Córdova, K. Vega, A. Chung, A. Villena, C. Góñez, and S. Castillo. "Effect of *Lepidium meyenii* (Maca) on Sexual Desire and Its Absent Relationship with Serum Testosterone Levels in Adult Healthy Men." *Andrologia* 34, no. 6 (December 2002): 367–372. https://pubmed.ncbi.nlm.nih.gov/12472620/.

INDEX

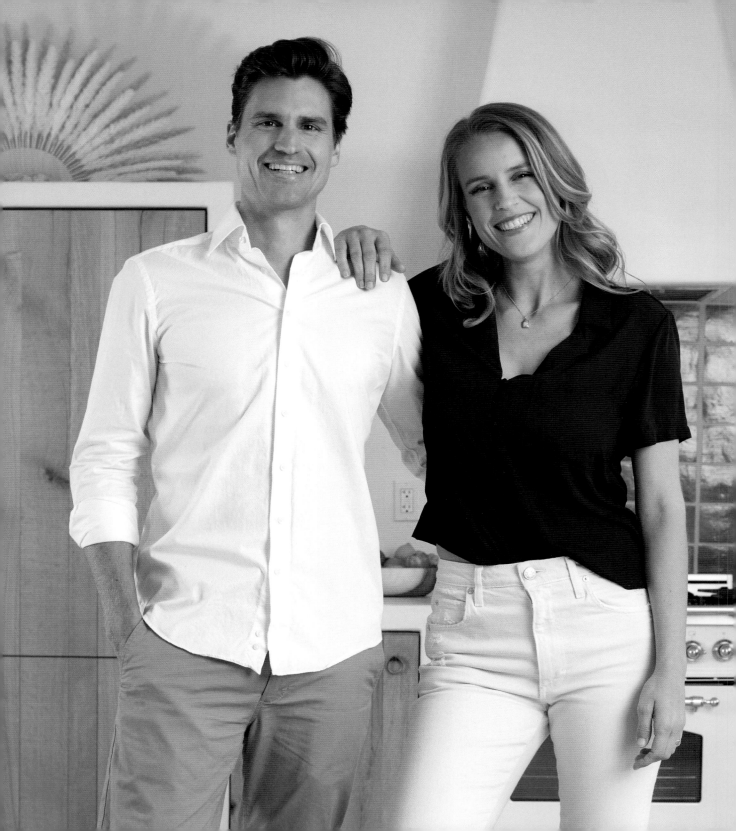

ABOUT THE AUTHORS

Kristel de Groot and **Michael Kuech** are cofounders of Your Super—a B Corp company that is on a mission to improve people's health with the power of super plants.

When Michael was 24, he was diagnosed with cancer. During his recovery Kristel helped boost his immunity with superfoods and a plant-based eating plan. Together they started Your Super—superfood mixes, plant-based proteins, organic snacks, online content, and a thriving community.

In the years since then they have gone from two people in Kristel's kitchen to an international community of more than a million. They committed to a transparent supply chain, working with small farmers, and creating the cleanest functional superfood mixes for everyday health, detoxing, immunity, hormone health, and gut support.

This duo have been featured on TV shows like *The Doctors*, *Good Day LA*, and the Cheddar streaming network and in publications like *People*, *Real Simple*, *Well + Good*, *Mind, Body, Green*, *InStyle*, *Yahoo Finance*, *Parade*, and others. Kristel was recognized as one of the *Forbes* 30 Under 30, and *Inc.*'s Rising Stars, while Michael is a sought-after speaker with a prolific Tedx Talk: "Is one of the biggest threats to humanity what is on our plates?"

Kristel holds a BBA in finance and accounting from Valdosta State University and an MSc in Management from Cass Business School, London. She received her certification in plant-based nutrition from eCornell University, graduated from Institute for Integrative Nutrition (IIN) as a plant-based health coach, has completed her 200-hour yoga teaching training, and is a former tennis pro. Michael was a consultant for Deutsche Bank, Ernst & Young, and more. He holds a BBA in finance and management from Valdosta State University, and MSc in finance from EBS Business School in Germany.

Michael and Kristel currently reside in Los Angeles and wherever their farmers have an extra hammock. They were recently married and have welcomed their first mini plant lover, a baby boy, who makes them extra appreciative for all the superfood support!

You can keep up with them on top-ranking **Your Super Podcast**, their site **kristelandmichael.com**, and on social **@kristelandmichael**.

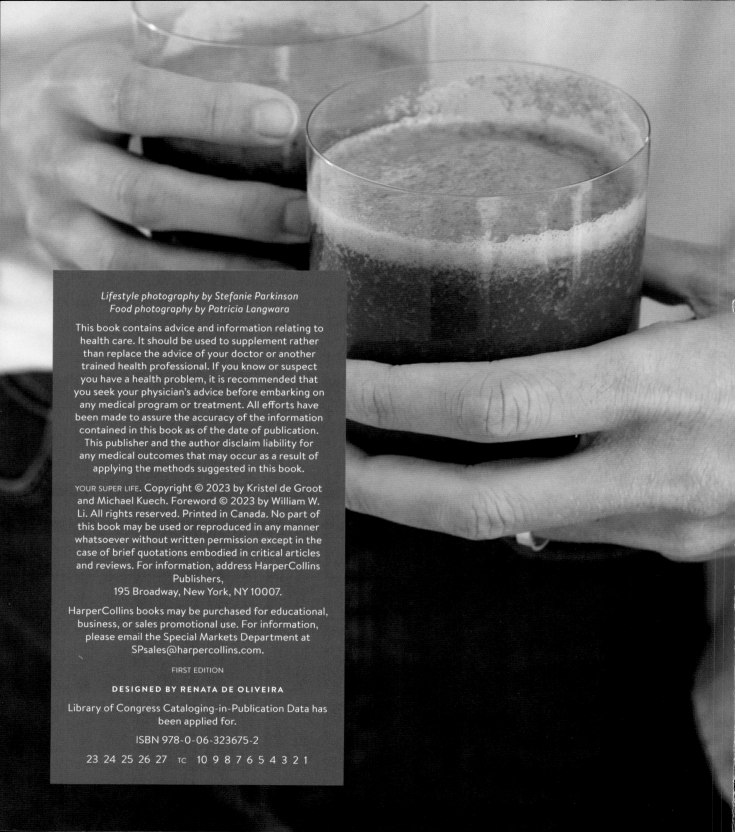

Lifestyle photography by Stefanie Parkinson
Food photography by Patricia Langwara

HarperCollins books may be purchased for educational, business, or sales promotional use. For information, please email the Special Markets Department at SPsales@harpercollins.com.

FIRST EDITION

DESIGNED BY RENATA DE OLIVEIRA

Library of Congress Cataloging-in-Publication Data has been applied for.

ISBN 978-0-06-323675-2

23 24 25 26 27   TC   10 9 8 7 6 5 4 3 2 1